Can[illegible]
Just a Bully

It Cannot Function in a Healthy Environment

The true story of one woman's victory over aggressive breast cancer without surgery or radiation.

An inspiration to anyone dealing with cancer or any degenerative disease.

Laurie Dunford

Cancer is Just a Bully
It Cannot Function
in a Healthy Environment

by Laurie Dunford

Laura B. Dunford, Publisher
Cover design and layout by Joseph Kennedy
Printed at Priority Printing Ltd., Edmonton, Alberta
November 2004, 1st Edition.

Dunford, Laurie, 1954-
Cancer is Just a Bully : It Cannot Survive in a
Healthy Environment / Laurie Dunford

Includes bibliographical references & Index.

ISBN #0-9736091-0-9

1. Cancer – Alternative Treatments
I. Title

RC270.8.D8522004 616.99'406 C2004-906788-5

Acknowledgments

I would like to thank Valerie Taylor for editing this book. I wish you tremendous success in your writing career.

Joseph Kennedy, thank you for doing the cover design and the formatting. You are very talented. I also wish you success and happiness.

How can I ever thank my mom enough? You have been there through everything.

Teresa and Jared Baudin, you made my garden look beautiful when I didn't have the energy.

Stewart Cooper, you were an angel of God, coming for an entire year and making carrot juice.

Louise Miller and Mars Hill Centre, you are always there for those who are hurting.

Allison Plishka, you were there every week to pray for me and listen to me.

Kim Ward, Dr. Vazquez, and all the staff at Sanovin Medical Institute, without you I don't believe I would be alive today. You gave me hope and strength to fight against incredible odds. It was wonderful to live in Paradise.

Dr. Lorraine Day, I've never met you but I can't thank you enough for all of your videos. You were a shining star in my dark night.

Rudy and Jeanie Davis, you are doing an awesome work in Lavoy Alberta.

Henrietta DeJong, how many times did you pick me up when I was falling apart?

Dr. George Malkmus, your book gave me such joy. I will spread your message everywhere: *"You Don't Have to be Sick!"*

Countless other people have helped me, and I thank you all.

Finally, the person I want to thank the most is my Saviour Jesus Christ who died that I might have life. Jesus you forgive all my sins and healed all my diseases. My life belongs to You and I will go where you lead me.

Contents

Introduction

This book is packed full of information that will help anyone dealing with cancer or other degenerative diseases. You will see the transformation in the author as she learns more about the causes of disease and its prevention. As she learns, you will learn. The book is written in diary style so the reader can walk along with her in pursuit of health and wellness. It is the intent of the author that you will have a life changing experience, just as she did. This book is well researched with over 45 references to experts in the fields of conventional and complementary medicine.

The book's central message is that cancer is not something that has to be feared. With the proper information, it is possible to prevent and reverse cancer. The problem is that the general population is not given all the information they need and neither do they receive it when they go to the doctor. The doctors are just as much in the dark as the patients they are treating! Much of what the author learned was contrary to what the conventional system puts forth. Her dramatic recovery has been a mystery to her doctors who told her she would die without the scientifically proven methods of surgery and radiation. She was ultimately healed by the Creator of the universe and the Creator of science itself. He is the One who knows what the body needs to heal itself. Much of what poses as science now-a-days is created by drug companies that do not want you to know the information in this book!

Enjoy this refreshing approach to overcoming a disease that is needlessly ravaging our population. Almost everyone knows someone who has cancer or another degenerative disease. After you read this book, you will understand that they do not have to be sick!

My Diagnostic Nightmare

I had my first chemotherapy treatment 11 days ago. I came home from work yesterday and slept for 12 hours. The Oncologist tells me that my hair will likely fall out in 10 more days. The wig is ready for that day when I wake up to my hair on the pillow. It is now March 24, 2001 and breast cancer in women is not decreasing, it is increasing. I was just diagnosed on March 5, 2001 and my disease is already at stage three (out of four). How could this happen? I was going for regular checkups, did breast self-examinations and informing the doctors of the changes I was noticing in my right breast. This question lead me to do considerable research on breast cancer diagnoses and treatment. What I am finding out does not put a favourable light on the doctors responsible for my diagnoses.

In January of 2000, I felt a distinctly solid lump at the 9 o'clock position and another one at the 11 o'clock position in my right breast. If you imagine the breast as a clock, that puts the lumps on the outside aspect of the breast, with the 11 o'clock lump being close to the armpit. In addition to the lumps, my breast felt quite a bit thicker on the underside and around the nipple. My doctor could feel it also, so I was sent for a mammogram. I have since learned that mammograms are only about 80-85 per cent effective in premenopausal women and their effectiveness is also dependent on the age of the machine. My mammogram came back normal in the right breast. I was then sent for an ultrasound on Jan 13, 2000, which showed a solid six mm mass at 9 o'clock and another six mm solid mass at 11 o'clock. The radiologist reported it as "likely benign but any decision to biopsy should be based on clinical criteria." The reason that he reported it like that, I have learned, is that "The general features of benign and malignant lesions have been established, but unfortunately many lesions do not conform to these 'classic descriptions'." (p963, Kopans et al, The New England Journal of Medicine, 1984)[1] In other words, the possibility of malignancy existed.

However, I was told by my family doctor that my ultrasound was normal and my lump was just a fibroadenoma. She never mentioned to me that there can be an overlap of some benign and malignant characteristics and the possibility of cancer still existed. I was not offered the choice to biopsy. Unfortunately, I thought she knew what she was doing.

Now I know from my research that "any new or previously unevaluated breast mass in any woman of any age that has a 'dominant' character must undergo biopsy without delay." (p223, Haskell,C.M. and Casciato,D.A., Breast Cancer, 2000)[2] I kick myself for trusting her and for not demanding a biopsy. "You may find that sometimes physicians and other health care providers, in their efforts not to alarm women, suggest that a lump is "probably nothing." The more sensitive and less damaging observation would be, "There is a lump in your breast. A biopsy will reveal whether the lump is cancerous or not." (p72, Cancer Stories on Life and Suffering, Dr. David M. Gregory, Dr. Cynthia K Russell)[3]

Breast cancers do not just show up overnight. "The average breast cancer requires 10 years or more to grow from a single cell to one cm, the size at which it can be readily detected by most patients or physicians." (p1884, Hematology and Oncology, Henderson,C.)[4] Factors which are known to contribute to breast cancer are: not having children, family history (in 10 per cent of cases), age (older than 40 years), and epidemiological evidence points strongly to the influence of diet in the pathogenesis of breast cancer. In other words fat is bad news. As much as I detest our western diet, I live in this society and my body has grown progressively larger over the last 10 years. In 1990 I weighed 145 lbs. When I was diagnosed I weighed 185 lbs. There has been a huge increase in the size of my breasts in the past five years. I've gone from a 36B to a 40F. When you look at all these factors, the only one I do not have is a family history. My body was screaming that I was a candidate for breast cancer.

In July 2000, I could still feel the lump, and the ultrasound was repeated. The mass was still there, "unchanged in size but now 'appears' cystic." Again I was glibly told that the test was normal. My breast still had thickenings along the outer and under side and again I was reassured that my breast was normal. By this time, I was beginning to wonder if there was even any use reporting the changes I noticed.

In October, my right nipple started to invert. I decided to go to a breast specialist and another mammogram was scheduled for December 1, 2000. Nothing showed. Again I was not informed that mammograms are often falsely negative in premenopausal women. An ultrasound showed "mild duct ectasia" on the right breast. This was explained to me as a deformity in the ducts, which was causing debris to build up and that was why my nipple was inverting. I was not told at this time that most breast cancers start in the ducts and then spread to the surrounding tissue. No other differential diagnoses was given to me and I was reassured that I "checked out" OK. My research revealed that over 80 per cent of breast cancers start in the ducts. Why did my doctor not do a biopsy? Now I was wondering not only what was the point of reporting these changes but what was the point of even looking for them. I had this false sense of security for 3 months. Then the bomb dropped.

The specialist recalled me on February 23, 2001. She examined my breast, then she frantically ran over to the radiologist and set up another mammogram and ultrasound. Meanwhile I sat and waited, knowing something was drastically wrong. She called me into her office and informed me that I had cancer throughout most of my breast and that it had probably spread throughout my body. I wondered why you would wait three months to re-examine an inverted nipple, especially if you could go from being normal and then three months later having cancer throughout your body.

Apparently this is the protocol in Alberta, although the literature says that an inverted nipple should be rechecked after the next menstrual cycle. What about just using common sense? Does technology rule over common sense? I spent the weekend paralyzed with fear that cancer may have spread throughout my body.

February 26, 2001 was my "emergency" biopsy. This should have been done a year ago. Most of my friends could not believe that this was really happening to me. My fear was real because I knew something had been dreadfully wrong for a long, long time. The specialist finally gave me the results on March 5, 2001. My biopsy was positive. I would be going to the Cross Cancer Institute for more tests, chemotherapy, and then I would be getting a bilateral mastectomy, followed by radiation, she said. She explained nothing to me about the kind of breast cancer I had or that I would even have any choices in my treatment. Again I was filled with panic. My long time friend Barb took me out for supper and talked and prayed with me for hours to calm me down. Rivotril, a pill to aid relaxation, was essential if I was going to get any sleep at all that night. I felt I was living with a death sentence, which was coming 40 years too early, and I did not want this to happen to any other woman. I needed to transform my anger into something positive by writing and informing others. Then I felt at least my suffering would not be in vain.

One evening towards the end of March 2001, I was lying on my bed paralyzed with fear and my friend Dina called. She invited me over for dinner on Monday March 26. While I was there Dina gave me a book called *Christ the Healer* by FF Bosworth.[5] I soaked up every word. I can honestly say that I have not suffered from fear since. It is the best exposition of the biblical scriptures on healing that I have ever read, and I've been a Christian for 25 years. Soon after, I attended a Healing conference in Abbotsford, B.C. where I was prayed for.

It is now April 19, 2001 and it is really easy to wash my hair because I do not have any. Another bonus is I do not have to shave my legs or my armpits. Yeah! My friends say my wig looks better than my previous hairstyle. Before I had my second chemotherapy two weeks ago, the Oncologist told me that he could no longer feel the swollen lymph nodes in my armpit. This was considered a good response to the first treatment. He had explained to me that my cancer was called inflammatory breast cancer. It had become so advanced that it had attached itself to the inner lining of my skin. It was pulling on the skin, giving it a peau d'orange or orange peel appearance. My breast looks all puckered and dimpled. Only 1-2% of breast cancers are this serious, and before the advent of chemotherapy, nobody ever survived inflammatory breast cancer (according to statistics). If I respond to the chemo, which it seems I am, I have a 90 per cent chance of surviving five years. If I don't respond, I will only have a 30 per cent chance of surviving five years (according to statistics).

Now it's Tuesday, April 24, 2001. I was supposed to get my chemo tomorrow but I cannot because my neutrophil count is too low. The treatment is rescheduled for Thursday. I got more books from the cancer institute library written by cancer survivors. I read a flow chart 'From discovery of a lump to diagnoses' from one of these books called "Breast Cancer, What You Should Know (But May Not Be Told)". It says that if a solid lump is found on the ultrasound aspiration cytology should be considered. (p12, Austiand Hitchcock, 1994)[6] My doctor did not discuss this consideration with me. This failure to biopsy puzzles me to no end. Even when I questioned the breast specialist why she didn't biopsy when the duct ectasia showed up, she said that she would be doing a lot of damage to women if she biopsied everything that was suspicious. My mom and my friend also heard her say that. It seems to me that it's a harmless procedure that can *prevent* a lot of serious damage. I would have preferred to have been diagnosed at stage one rather than stage three. I spoke to the radiologist in March 2001 about why he was not more insistent on a biopsy when he saw the solid lump on the ultrasound. He told me something that totally baffled me. He said that doctors who order too many biopsies are taken out of the screening program. That has raised a lot of questions in my mind. Who makes these decisions that a doctor has done too many biopsies? Why is a doctor taken out of a screening program for doing "too many" prophylactic biopsies? I want to talk to the people who make these decisions.

It is Saturday, April 28, 2001. I just received a phone call from a friend of mine who is a family practitioner in the city. I gave him an update on my progress and recapped the diagnostic history. He also is baffled by the failure to biopsy. He thought that if something new and suspicious showed up on a screening test that you were supposed to take it out and look at it. He also said that at some point somebody is going to have to sit down with me and tell me honestly that they goofed and failed me in a huge way. Actually, the breast specialist did admit to me in March 2001 that clearly there had to have been cancer in my breast back in December 2000, and she missed it. My mother and my friend Barb both heard her say that. I had to ask the breast specialist a lot of questions before she actually reluctantly admitted it.

I need all the information I can get, but I still believe it is God who is going to heal me. Focusing on scriptures has the most positive effect on me. It's Saturday May 5, 2001. I have just returned from a conference session with Dr. Randy White from Florida. He talked about how we need to take a step towards God before He will take a step towards us. He also taught that being a conqueror does not mean we never get knocked down, it means we get up after we get knocked down, and we keep fighting. He used an illustration from a boxing match of a champion who was knocked down and almost out, but got up and went on to win the fight. That is going to be me. I am knocked down right now but I'm going to keep believing. Today I slept most of the day, but I was ready to do battle with the enemy tonight and we really gave him some bad punches. I feel full of joy so Satan cannot be very happy right now. My friend Joyce told me tonight about her healing from an adrenal tumor back in the late '80s. The doctors did not have to operate because the tumor disappeared! This beautiful native lady now spends much of her time in intercessory prayer for others. I am encouraged!

Now it is Sunday May 6, 2001. I have processed some information that I got from a book at the Cross Cancer Institute. I quote Dr. Susan Love the breast specialist: "...anyone with a lump needs to have it biopsied regardless of the mammogram." (p173,*My Breast*, Wadler,J.;1992)[7] I think my ex-family doctor needs to read that. On the same page of the same book, Dr. Susan Love goes on to say: "The problem is that most cancers have been there a long time by the time we find them. The average cancer has a doubling time of 100 days; it takes 100 days for one cell to double and become two. You need 100 billion cancer cells to have one centimetre of cancer. If you do the math, you'll see that most cancers have been present for eight or ten years by the time you can feel the smallest of lumps. A long time." I did the math. If my tumor was 11 cm at the end of Feb/01, as they said it was, it would have contained 1 trillion, 100 billion cancer cells. If you calculate back to Jan/00, it would have contained about 68 billion cancer cells and been about 6mm, which is exactly what showed up on the ultrasound - a six mm. solid lump. In that year that they kept a watch on it, it doubled from 6 mm. to 1.2 cm., then from 1.2 cm. to 2.4 cm., then from 2.4 cm. to 4.8, and from 4.8 cm, to 9.6 cm. My point is that when something keeps doubling like that, waiting a year to "see what it does" is stupid, irresponsible, and incomprehensible. Add to that the fact that not only were cancer cells spreading from the ducts on the lateral aspect of my breast they were spreading from the ducts on the inferior aspect as well. An invasion was going on all over my breast, yet I was told by the breast specialist in December 2000 that the lumps throughout my breast were normal. Not once did she or my family doctor ever tell me that cancer is usually present for about 10 years before it shows as a 1 cm. lump. I have equal years of post-secondary education to a doctor, do they think I'm incapable of understanding this, or is it that they want to keep a mystique around it, thus increasing their sense of power? The average woman with a high school education is capable of understanding this, so why aren't we told? My whole purpose in life is to empower others so they can live a full life as God intended, so I don't understand people who want to keep people ignorant.

A whole month has past since I last wrote in here. It is June 5, 2001. I received the investigative report from the College of Physicians and Surgeons last week. Apparently they do not find anything wrong with a doctor leaving a solid lump or an inverted nipple unbiopsied. God have mercy on the 20 out of 100 women whose benign-looking malignant lumps are not biopsied. I sent back a response and asked them to reinvestigate. They tried to tell me that this cancer was insidious and just snuck up on me with no warning. I was complaining for a year and a half, so it was hardly "insidious". It gets so hard for me to take that on days when I have a lot of pain. The last couple of chemo treatments do not seem to have made much difference in the tumor. The doctors can not guarantee that microscopic cancer cells will not be floating around in my system after the chemo, the mastectomy and the radiation are all done. There has to be another way to treat this.

I felt I had to increase my odds. A friend had told me about a herbal supplement called Oncolyn a few months ago, so I gave the distributor a call yesterday. I picked up the pills and talked to her for a good hour. Several people who have taken it have had their cancer disappear, even without conventional treatment. Sherry, the distributor, felt that God had lead her to this product to help her son, who had testicular cancer which had spread to other areas of his body. He's fine today and is a recent father. Her faith was unwavering that her son was going to live and she didn't stop looking until she found something that worked. I'm not going to stop believing either.

Since I last wrote, I had my fifth chemo treatment on June 13, 2001. That one completely zapped me of strength. I slept for days and nights on end and could accomplish only one or two things a day, like meeting a friend for dinner and then going home and back to bed. This had a very depressive effect on me. After about a week I started to come out of it and I was able to go to the market and grocery store with my boyfriend, Allan, on Saturday. Allan had come across an interesting book called *Eating Right For Your Type* by Dr. D'Adamo, a naturopathic doctor. His basic concept is that certain foods are beneficial to specific blood types and other foods can be toxic to that same blood type.[8] I'm a Type A, and meat is not recommended for my type. This made a lot of sense to me, because I usually do not feel great after I eat meat. He also stated that epidemiological evidence shows that Type A's are more prone to breast cancer and more frequently have relapses. This means that world-wide Type A's fare more poorly with respect to this type of cancer. Armed with that information, he gives ammunition as to how one can increase his/her odds of survival. I found the book to be revolutionary and devoured it in a couple of days. Since he's already tested the effects of different foods on different blood types, I made a copy of the foods I should and should not be eating. Apricots are now a wonderful addition to my diet, as is soy milk.

A few days after Allan lent me the book on blood types, my friend Teresa lent me a book by Jane A Plant Ph.D. called *Your Life in Your Hands.* Dr. Plant is a five-time survivor of breast cancer, and the last time she had a relapse, in 1993, the doctors told her she only had three to six mos. to live. She realized that surgery, chemotherapy, and radiation had not saved her life and began to look for the root cause of the cancer. This is what has been bothering me about the medical establishment, is that no one seems interested in even looking at possible causes.

Instead they appear more interested in following treatment protocols. When I told my oncologist that this Ph.D. scientist had treated herself successfully by making serious changes in her diet, he was not even interested to know more about it. Dr. Plant has scientific evidence for all of her conclusions but he doesn't even want to look at it. She is also a highly esteemed scientist in Britain and won Britain's most prestigious science honor in 1999, the Lord Lloyd of Kilgerran Prize. Other recipients of this award include the inventor of the World Wide Web and the inventor of DNA fingerprinting.

What Dr. Plant had to say has completely changed my life. While it has long been known that women from China have drastically lower rates of breast cancer than North American women, and that their rates go up when Chinese women move to the west, I have never seen such definitive evidence for the dietary cause before. I thought it had something to do with the amount of soy they eat, but I didn't think that the thing they don't eat also protects them. What do they not eat that we do? The answer is dairy products. They think cows milk is for cows, and they can not understand our preoccupation with milk, cheese, yogurt, ice cream and numerous other dairy products.

After I read all the chapters about the chemicals and hormones in milk, I got rid of my milk, yogurt and cheese and ordered soy milk through home delivery. I was amazed! I like it better than the skim milk that I had been faithfully drinking for decades! I looked through my "eating right for your type" lists of food and found that milk is a definite food to avoid for people with type A blood. It's been a few days since I weaned myself, and I've noticed that the tumor is softening up even more and getting smaller. Don't forget it was 11cm. by 9 cm.! Without going into great detail about the hormones involved, I would have to say, read the book, because she has done an unbelievable amount of research. Genetically engineered bovine growth hormone (BGH), and insulin-like growth factor (IGF-1) are only two of many chemicals that are of concern. Dr. Plant found out that she was not the first person to advise breast cancer patients to avoid death by dairy. There is a Dr. R.M. Kradjian, M.D. from Daly City California, who had come to similar conclusions and has written a book called *Save Yourself From Breast Cancer.*[9] When I went on the Internet, I found 45,000 articles relating to dairy and breast cancer. I can't wait till I have time to wade through them. I'm very thankful to the Holy Spirit who I believe led my two friends to these books. Christians from various churches have come over every Tuesday for almost four months to pray for answers to our cry for healing.

My Sanoviv Experience

At the beginning of July, 2001 I made a drastic decision to go against my oncologist's recommendation. He told me that going to a clinic in Mexico would not be beneficial to me. He was not familiar with Sanoviv and had no interest in listening to anything I had to say about it. After making a joke about me turning orange from drinking carrot juice, he said it probably would not do me any damage, but it would not do me any good either. His plan was to do surgery within 3 weeks. No reconstruction would be possible because the kind of breast cancer I have is aggressive and often grows back in the chest wall. In other words, surgery would not necessarily take care of the problem! After stating that, he proceeded to make an appointment with the surgeon, which turned out to be 5 weeks down the road! I figured if I had to wait 5 weeks to see the surgeon anyway, what difference would it make if I went to Mexico for two weeks in between? Most of my friends were supportive of me going to Sanoviv and all of the people I know from working with the Usana Nutritional Company were highly recommending it. With their encouragement I decided to go. I wish I had gone sooner.

One of the first things I learned in Sanoviv is that doctors, naturopaths, psychologists, colon hydrotherapists, massage therapists, spa therapists, nurses and dieticians can work together. I arrived on Sunday, July 15, 2001 and on Monday morning, July 16, all the department heads met to discuss my case and decide their plan of attack against the illnesses within me. Each member of the treatment team knew what the other members were doing. It was recognized that all the disciplines had something to offer and that no single treatment would kill this cancer. Praise God! There was no egoism, no scoffing, no put downs, only a united effort to kill the beast. A positive treatment team is needed when you're dealing with cancer.

What I learned at Sanoviv is powerful ammunition for those who choose to actively participate in their healing process. I am still assimilating all the healthy choices I learned into my lifestyle. There are a few people who remain sceptical of what I am doing, but not many. Nobody can argue with the fact that I look much healthier than before I went to Sanoviv. I lost fifteen pounds while

I was there and another five when I came back. I still have a minimum of 20 lbs. to go but I feel confident I can do it with the dietary information I received. Most of all my spirit is up.

Since I was in treatment from 7 a.m. till 8 or 9 p.m., I was not always able to write in my journal. I do have my daily schedules so I know exactly what I was doing everyday. I want to explain all the treatments to the best of my ability so that others can learn from my experience.

July 16,2001 was the first treatment day. I awoke naturally at 6:30 a.m. I had to take saliva and urine samples to the lab and have blood taken. One of the things the doctors are testing for is the Ph level. If the urine is too alkaline it can mean that the tissues are acidic, and this kind of environment or bio-terrain, is not good. If your Ph is balanced, it is easier to fight off the cancer cells. At the fitness evaluation my body fat turned out to be 39 per cent - a very poor result, but not unexpected. I knew the fitness classes were going to be crucial to my healing. We had sprouts for lunch and then surprisingly we had sprouts for supper! I just about burnt my mouth on the radish sprouts! It was a shock to learn that sprouts and raw vegetables were to be the mainstay of all our lunches and suppers. Millet, quinoa or fruit was for breakfast.

July 17, 2001 was a fun day as far as treatments. I had a Swedish massage, a manicure and facial. I entered the following in my journal: Today I slept in even though sunlight was streaming through my window. We have no curtains here so we can wake up naturally. I am still taking rivotril so I don't wake up that easily. I missed fitness class and getting my vitals taken. Every morning before 7 a.m. we are expected at the nursing station to get weighed, and have our blood pressure, heart rate and oxygen levels taken. The nurses told me they missed me this morning. I did make it to meditation at 8 a.m. That is run by the psychology department. For our meditation we thought about different people we knew and prayed for blessing on their lives.

After breakfast I had a consultation with Dr. Vazquez who is a very thorough doctor. I like him because he has a feisty personality and wants to work with me to beat this cancer. He's putting me on some biological immune stimulators and modulators. One is Pind-avi, which is capable of producing activation of the immune system, another, Eurixor (Mistletoe), will be injected into the borders of the tumor once we build up the dose. Mistletoe is widely used in Europe. Dr. Vazquez is also administering some orthomolecular supplementation. One of the supplements is called Wobe-Mugus, which kills the cancer cells from the inside out. Dr. Vazquez is also giving an Isopathic treatment every Monday, Wednesday and Friday - in the evenings I get an injection of Sanuvis and in the mornings, an injection of Pleo-muc. These treatments are new to me so I am writing them all down to help me learn them. I also have a homeopathic treatment with Cantharis drops three times/day. This is only a sampling of what is being done. He emphasized everyone's treatment is individually tailored to their needs. As patients we shouldn't compare therapies.

On the 18th, the third day of therapy, I started thalasso pool treatments. There are three of these salt-water pools at Sanoviv. One is hot (about 104 degrees), the other is about body temperature, and the other is cold. We spend about 20 minutes walking around in the hot pool and a lesser amount of time in the other pools. I feel totally relaxed when I am in the hot pool. Sea salt is thought to be very therapeutic for cancer patients.

I gave myself my first enema tonight after listening to a detox lecture by Maggie. We are supposed to do them every night except on days when we have a colonic scheduled. They found I have a malabsorption problem. That means I have a build up of old mucus and debris on the walls of my intestines and I am lacking certain digestive enzymes. This can be due to a number of things but dairy products are definitely contributing because they found out I am actually allergic to them. Here I have been faithfully drinking my milk for 47 years so I would not get osteoporosis and I have been doing more harm than good. Guess what? Not one dairy product is served at Sanoviv.

On July 19, 2001 I wrote that I just had a wonderful spa treatment. Spa therapies are very helpful to cancer patients but they are not offered as part of our conventional treatment nor do the doctors recommend that we go to a spa. Over the course of the three weeks I was there I had many different treatments. One time, I was painted with seaweed and wrapped up for 20 minutes. Another time I was put in a hot pool with volcanic ash and I sweated profusely. This helps remove toxins from the body. The spa therapists were extremely well trained. I know now what to look for when I seek someone in my area.

The naturopath, Oliver, did extensive testing on the Vega equipment and he found I had high levels of lead, palladium and mercury in my body. These heavy metals contribute to a weakening of the immune system. I have eight lovely mercury fillings in my mouth and I am sure I had more in the past that were replaced with white fillings. The chelation therapy I had lowered the amounts of lead and palladium but it does not lower the mercury counts. I have been able to find someone in Edmonton, Henrietta, who does Vega testing and Vega therapy. This is a Godsend because there are few places in Canada that perform the testing and therapy.

Some of the other therapies I found helpful at Sanoviv were Rife therapy, Photon Laser Therapy, Infrared heat therapy and Matrix Regeneration Therapy (MRT). I found none of these therapies are offered in Edmonton at this time. I do have a very good massage therapist and colon hydrotherapist all in one person, Sharon. She goes the extra mile for her patients.

Twice a day at 11 a.m. and 4 p.m. at Sanoviv we were given fresh squeezed vegetable juice. My particular blend was carrot, beet and blueberry. Also at 10 a.m. and 3 p.m. we had a couple of ounces of fresh wheatgrass. One ounce of wheatgrass equals a couple of pounds of green leafy vegetables. To get the full benefit of wheatgrass you should not eat or drink anything one half hour before or after drinking it. Here, at home I am a regular customer at Booster Juice. However, I only get a juice about every second day and a wheatgrass about once a week, so the therapeutic effect is not as intense. My goal is to eventually get a good juicer and do it myself. I was advised at Sanoviv to give the biological medicine at least three months to work and then reconsider the possibility of surgery. I was given: Indole 3-carbinol, which is a cruciferous extract, and is known to prevent cancer, Samyr and milk thistle to help detox the liver, mistletoe which has anti-tumor properties, liv-uno or artichoke extract, calcium D-glucarate, wobe mugos (an enzyme), decaris, Proflavanol C (grapeseed extract), and the Essentials (multiminerals and antioxidants).

The doctors at Sanoviv also wanted me to take Gemzar, a chemotherapy agent, at the same time, to prevent metastases. This is not normally given in Alberta for breast cancer and is not covered by the Alberta Health Care system. However my oncologist here did agree to give me Taxotere, which is a much stronger agent than Gemzar. It also has strong side effects that I was not prepared for. The list of side effects includes muscle and joint pain, but the list does not say that this can be severe. Several days after my first dose I was convinced I had bone metastases because I was in so much pain. I found out from one of the doctors where I work who is an oncologist, that some people find taxotere so excruciating that they discontinue it. Once I knew that I could cope with it better, but it would have been nice to know ahead of time.

The pain curtailed any plans I had for excercise, which was disappointing to me. I had started a TaI ChI class and I just couldn't make it every week. It also had a depressive affect on me, so my friend Allison asked some people if I could come over for meals. I did not even have the energy to make the phone calls so it was nice of her to do that. At this point of writing it's Oct 27, 2001. I've had 3 doses of taxotere and have one more to go in mid-November. Then we do an MRI (Magnetic Resonance Imaging) to see if there is anything still in the right breast.

On October 23, 2001, I watched a video by Dr. Lorraine Day called *Cancer Doesn't Scare Me Anymore*. Dr. Day had a huge breast tumor in 1993 leading her to implement a 10-step natural treatment plan without the use of chemotherapy, radiation and surgery. She said once she began following the plan her cancer was gone in 10 months. This plan was similar to what was included in the Sanoviv program. Dr. Day recommended: a vegan diet; juicing, exercise; devotional time; no toxic substances such as sugar, coffee, aspartame or alcohol; lots of water; fresh air; sunlight; an attitude of gratitude; a spirit of benevolence, and proper rest.

Something else that Dr. Day said is essential to healing is dealing with resentment and anger. Sanoviv has an excellent psychology department. I met with Kim several times per week and we dealt a lot with my emotions. In Bernie Siegel's book, *Peace, Love and Healing*, which was in the library at Sanoviv, I read something that struck a chord deep within me. There was a study done on childhoods and future diseases and the researcher was surprised at the results: "...cancer patients, ...were much more likely than the other subjects in the study to ...have reacted by repressing their emotions in the years since" (p156)[11] In many ways I had a very privileged childhood and I am grateful for the many benefits I received. I was good in school, in music and in sports. When I was a teenager, some very bad things happened to me. After they happened, I wanted to die. I stopped playing music and sports. I tried to commit suicide. I've worked very hard to regain my self-esteem. Many cancer patients have a history of trauma.

The Learning Continues

Now it is November 18, 2001. It seems as if I am working towards a Masters Degree in How to Fight Cancer. The plethora of available information is unending. I've been following Dr. Lorraine Day's plan for three weeks now and I feel great! It is amazing how something as simple as fresh air, which God has provided, can make such a big difference in how you feel. I go for a walk every lunch break at work for half an hour. I always used to think I was stuck in my building all day. How our thinking limits us! Yesterday, Saturday, I went for a walk with my friend Renuka, which is a blessing for her because she is blind. So she gets a guide and we both get company. Today the sun was shining so brightly I just had to go out and rake some leaves. Since my neighbour was outside we began chatting. She's a medical student so I shared with her my dream that complementary medicinal practitioners and western trained doctors would one day work together in the same facilities. I told her I'm discovering so much from complementary medicine.

A few weeks ago, I started an immune booster made from Bovine Colostrum extract, arabinogalactan, Maitake mushroom extract and astragalus. The colostrum is from cows raised on an organic farm. I had almost no muscle pain from my last chemo treatment on Wednesday. Several people at church told me that I had my glow back. This product, called AG Immune, was developed by an immunologist in the States named Dr. Jesse Stoff. Dr. Stoff's research shows that natural killer cells, which are not functioning properly and are depleted in cancer patients can be triggered so that the person can better fight the disease. I certainly feel increased energy.

When I first saw the oncologist in March of this year he told me that if I responded to the chemotherapy I would have a 90% chance of surviving past 5 years, if I had the surgery and radiation after the chemo. If I did not respond I would only have a 30% chance. Because I responded - my tumor has shrunk to about half it's original size - I was thinking I had a good chance. But on Tuesday he clearly stated that it's only if you have no cancer cells at the time of surgery that you have such a high chance. Can you believe it? If I had gone into surgery in September as he was pushing me to do, with the tumor only down to six cm by four cm, I would have had a very low chance. The possibility of making it worse certainly existed. If the MRI last week is normal or close to normal, it seems to make sense to keep working on killing all the cancer cells. And if all the cancer cells are dead, what is the point of surgery? No wonder Dr.Vazquez at Sanoviv was so angry that the cancer institute was pushing me into surgery without giving me any other options.

Today, November 19, 2001 after a totally satisfying supper of organic spinach and organic brown rice I'm settling down for another writing session. I stopped at the library after work to do more internet research and found that there is a huge amount of information on natural killer cells and cancer. I think I'm on the right track by taking the AG Immune product. Since chemotherapy destroys most of the natural killer cells it ironically leaves you less able to fight off any comeback by the cancer, therefore building the natural killer cells back up is crucial. Many patients relapse after treatment so it seems wise to take this precaution, especially because I have the most aggressive form of breast cancer.

I awoke a bit late today, November 21, 2001 and immediately the hunter-gatherer went into gear. I hadn't prepared anything for breakfast, so as soon as I got a break at work I was down at the organic store searching for grains and vegetables. Popping the instant oatmeal into the microwave is no longer allowed! I got a whole bag of organic lettuce for lunch - it is cheaper than buying a restaurant prepared salad. Yesterday, I craved fruit so I went hunting for berries at the grocery store. A blended fruit drink before supper - nothing better!

On Friday, November 23, I saw a lymphologist. The tech worked on unblocking my lymphatic and ileocecal valves. It is interesting that the lymphatic valve is on the right, just below the collar bone. The majority of breast lumps in women occur on the right breast. I thought that something must not be working right in there but I did not under-stand the physiology. No doctor has even told me about my lymphatic valve. It seems to be quite valuable information when one is dealing with breast cancer. I had never heard of lymphology before, but this person studied it in Germany. When his wife became ill and conventional medicine offered no answers, he began searching the world. His wife is much healthier now, in her 60's, than she was in her 40's. I'm really impressed that a man would go to such lengths for the love of his wife. He could easily have resigned himself to an unhealthy situation as many people do.

Now it is the beginning of December. We have had tons of snow and lots of cold weather. It does not bother me at all because last week I got my MRI results and the doctor could not find the tumor! Of course the MRI does not show if microscopic cells are present so my excitement is contained. Most women do have cancer cells when the breast is removed and examined. Now I really need a second opinion, because my oncologist still wants to go ahead with the mastectomy. As the surgeon said, the treatment protocol as of this date, 2001 is chemo, surgery and radiation. As of 2002 the protocol could change. In fact, all indications are that it will change. They are telling me that if I don't have surgery within 3 months it will be too late to operate and I will die. Why do they pronounce these death sentences? There has to be a better way of dealing with this disease. I don't want to make a decision based on fear, I want to make one based on God, although I do have a healthy fear of this enemy. As Dr. Lorraine Day says, "You Can't Improve on God".[12]

It turns out, the radiation oncologist read my MRI wrong and there still is cancer visible, likely in the ducts. This news was delivered by the surgeon I saw on December 3, 2001. That was a very upsetting day. I called Dr. Vazquez down in Sanoviv and he suggested coming back for two weeks in January. Immediately I felt peace about going. They are closed for Christmas until January 7, so I made plans to go when they reopen. Of course he cannot promise I'll be healed but he is willing to work with me to help eradicate the rest of the cancer cells. I'm looking forward to the non-toxic environment, being able to soak up some sunlight and to once again eat the Garden of Eden diet.

Friday, December 7, 2001 my friend Nick came over. He has been battling prostate cancer for over a year. He just found out that his PSA (prostate level) has returned to normal. Hooray! He gets a clean bill of health. Now he can go to Tibet to teach English as a Second Language. Not bad for a 69 year old man! God has shown Nick as He has shown me the importance of diet, exercise, having an attitude of gratitude, studying the Word of God, having a spirit of benevolence, and staying away from toxins. He gave me a book by Dr. Don Colbert, Benny Hinn's physician, called *The Bible Cure for Cancer.*[13] I soaked it up this weekend. I showed him and my friend Dina Dr. Day's video "You can't improve on God". Nick agreed you could not go wrong with Dr. Day's advice. His surgeon had really pushed him to have surgery when he was diagnosed, but Nick knew instinctively there had to be a better way. Now he's cancer free!

Since my chemo is over I have returned to injecting Mistletoe. Dr. Vazquez told me to ask the nurse to put half of the vial in the breast and half in the arm to prevent metastases. I have just enough vials to last until I go back to Mexico. When I returned to using mistletoe at the beginning of December I had a strong reaction initially. I became very tired, almost as tired as the chemo made me. My nurse at the alternative health clinic, Henrietta, explained this is a good sign because it means the mistletoe is working. I was not convinced in the beginning because it seemed to become more inflamed. However, now it has settled down and it is hard to find the tumor. Henrietta explained that the cancer knows it's being attacked and is going out fighting. Good analogy.

It was a beautiful sunny day today and there was no wind at all. It is December 22, 2001 and I just returned from a walk around the neighbourhood. Since I learned that fresh air is essential for healing from cancer, I try not to miss a day. If a person stays indoors all day he doesn't get enough of the right kind of ions, specifically negative ions created by sunlight reacting with the molecules in the air. Ironically, many cancer patients are kept inside all day and are denied the very thing they need for health. My daily walks seem to revitalize me and clear my head. I receive three bonuses in one-shot exercise, fresh air and life-sustaining sunlight.

The Christmas festivities are over and I managed to survive without gaining any weight. My mom, who has been a tremendous support throughout my entire ordeal, got me a juicer for Christmas. At my earliest opportunity, I went out and bought a 25 lb bag of organic carrots. It makes such sweet juice. Cleaning the juicer was not as bad as I thought it would be. My sister Jennifer had several of her in-laws over on Christmas day. All expressed interest in my new way of eating. Hugh, my brother, gave me a vegetarian cookbook, which was also popular with the guests. Jennifer bought me the book *Fit for Life* by Harvey and Marilyn Diamond. I have wanted to read *Fit for Life* for quite awhile because it was on the recommended reading list at Sanoviv. Health was definitely the theme this Christmas!

One of the gifts I gave to my friend Allison was the book *Sugar Blues* by William Dufty.[14] Allison was happy to receive this book, because sugar is the last remaining vice she is trying to kick. I bought myself a copy of the book and it really is an eye opener. William Dufty goes into the history of the sugar industry and shows the depths that refined sugar has infiltrated into most of our food products. How it contributes to diabetes is well known but all the other problems it creates are not common knowledge. It is amazing that sugar is considered to be a staple when it does not even have any nutritional value. Sugar is high in calories and has strong addictive properties. I know because I was addicted before I went to Sanoviv. I did not put on 50 lbs in 10 years because of the aging process!

Just after New Years I returned to Sanoviv. I have been back 2 weeks already. I went back to work immediately on my return and found it was hard to find time to write. My plane landed in Calgary, my sister's husband picked me up, I had supper with them and drove home that evening, arriving at almost midnight. The next morning, January 21, a snow storm blew in so I am glad I came when I did. For the last two weeks we have been in deep freeze temperatures. The idea that I have been hatching to live in Mexico got a lot stronger!

The first couple of days at Sanoviv there were only three patients, and one patient's husband. Sandy had lung cancer, and the other lady had a pituitary adenoma. We really felt well looked after! After two days of intensive testing the treatment team found

I had several main issues to be addressed. The dark field microscope showed proteolytic enzyme deficiency, chemical toxicity, liver stress, the presence of cholesterol and uric acid crystals, arthritis tendency, and lymphatic clogging. The Bio Terrain Assessment, the Vega test and the Diagnostic Functional Medicine (DFM) test, all showed lymphatic clogging. The DFM also revealed really low energy states in the upper part of the body. The consensus was that the high levels of mercury in my mouth were likely contributing to this, so I had two of my mercury fillings in the upper right quadrant removed.

My fitness evaluation was much better than when I was there in July. They were really pleased that I had kept my weight off and started walking everyday. Just walking for 30 minutes a day made a big difference. The proportion of lean body mass has gone up and the amount of body fat has gone down, but it is still poor. Ideally I should be another 35 lbs lighter at 125 lbs but 145 would do! Ricardo, one of the fitness instructors, was very encouraging. The fitness training is very gentle and is geared for people with compromised health. We used rebounders (mini-trampolines) and Swiss balls (for stretching) first thing in the morning for about 45 minutes. I sure did not see any rebounders or Swiss balls at the Cross Cancer Institute! They are not that expensive either!

I spoke to my oncologist here in Edmonton and informed him of the treatment I'm taking. He was quite upset that I had not gone for surgery, but he did admit that there could be some benefit to being on arimidex and UFT. He said whoever put me on Zoladex was crazy, but it works with the Arimidex, so Sanoviv's doctors had a good reason for what they did. Both drugs inhibit estrogen production and as my tumor is estrogen positive, the less estrogen it has to feed on the better. I had to remind my oncologist that my tumor was estrogen positive as he could not remember. He said a study was done on UFT and it does have an antitumor effect, but he's still concerned about metastases. While I do appreciate the concern, I cannot tell if he is angry because I'm listening to a Mexican and not to him or if he thought that by getting angry he could scare me into going for surgery. I am sure he's genuinely concerned because I'm outside of standard protocol, but I'm also concerned, and plan to have another MRI in a month to see if this therapy is working. If it's not working I will use the more drastic measures, but why get drastic right away? I do not think it was fair of him to tell me, "You're playing with your life." I think the cancer industry plays with peoples' lives all the time. Now he tells me that he's only had one other patient who refused surgery, only taking chemo and radiation, and she's still alive over 5 years later!

My oncologist also told me that I should get in for radiation right away, so he set me up to see the radiation specialist. She appeared very kind and did not judge me for my decisions. She even revealed to me that currently there is a study going on with arimidex, but only women with more common breast cancers can participate in it. Rare forms like inflammatory type do not qualify, consequently there is no information on how it responds. If I hadn't have gone to Mexico I would not have received arimidex. Apparently the study is showing very positive results - great tumor shrinkage. Dr. Vazquez says it produces positive results with inflammatory breast cancer, but his numbers are so small that they would be considered "anecdotal" by conservative doctors. I would sure like to be one of the "anecdotes"! Currently, the standard treatment for inflammatory cancer is based on the Anderson study (chemo, surgery, radiation) - 10 years from now it might be different. Even in two years it could change. That's how scientific "science" is!

February 11, 2002. I went to the oasis church yesterday to hear singer/songwriter Lianna Klassen. I love her *Song For Canada*. Sharon Sonnenberg was there and she is such an inspiration to me. Four years ago God healed her of lung tumors, metastasized from the breast. Now when I say God healed her, I don't mean that she didn't do her part. I was amazed to hear what she did. Went for walks everyday, drank carrot juice, ate fruits, vegetables, grains, read the Bible, meditated on scripture and listened to uplifting music. Sounds like Dr. Lorraine Day all over again, but Sharon said she had never heard of Lorraine Day. I do not know what else she did, but those are the things she told me.I guess she is considered to be an "anecdotal case" at the Cross Cancer Institue. No chemo, no surgery, no radiation, no cancer. How can it be? I told her how my doctor had scared me last week and she said, "whose report are you going to believe, the doctor's report or the report in this book?" (pointing to the bible) O.K! Now I am ready to do warfare again!

Now You're on Your Own

February 12, 2002. I've abandoned my essay style of writing for a diary style. At work today I had a really crabby patient. I decided to tell her I had cancer and she softened up a lot. She had been through breast cancer herself 10 years ago and could empathize. It's amazing how when you open up to people they really open up to you.

My boss, Dr. Tai, brought oranges and rice cakes for all us staff because it is Chinese New Year. The orange made a good breakfast because I did not get up in time to make anything. This is really my area of weakness right now and always has been. I had a student staying with me from Spain a few years ago and she got up every morning to go for a jog. Boy did I admire her. Some mornings I get up in time to do my rebounding. Kim, the psychotherapist at Sanoviv, gave me some positive affirmations to say to myself. One of them was "I have the self-discipline I need to keep on a healthy schedule." I need to start saying that to myself several times a day. Having acknowledged that, it is 9:30 so I am going to bed.

February 13, 2002. Made vegetarian stew for Allison. She loved it, so I was happy that I blessed someone today. We had a prayer time after. She is leaving for Ghana on a medical mission in a couple of weeks.

February 14, 2002. Met Louise for supper at the Two Rooms Café. They make great vegetarian burgers there. Had my abdominal ultrasound this afternoon and it was good news - normal organs! Louise has been a major support to me.

February 15, 2002. Worked this morning, and then went to the dental school in the afternoon. I have really got the dental student thinking about the whole mercury debate, because last week I refused to let them put in a mercury filling. I had to sign a statement saying that I understood white fillings do not last as long as "silver" fillings.

Just going off to meet Sheree for "coffee", which really means herbal tea. First I have to do the rebounding thing.

February 16, 2002. Terry came over for tea today then we went for a walk. Beautiful, sunny day. Belgravia is such a nice neighbourhood to walk in - so many trees. Terry was interested in my book, *Sugar Blues*, so I lent it to her.

Went for a body wrap after she left. The process is so relaxing I almost fell asleep. It sure didn't measure up to a Sanoviv spa treatment though.

February 17, 2002. Kim lent me her champion juicer today. Kim and Jim used it when their little guy was battling cancer. Lately, it was just collecting dust. (Their little boy has been OK for 2 years now.) Wow, a champion juicer! Now I can take my smaller one to work and have carrot juice a couple of times a day. Champion juicers were used down in Sanoviv and were highly recommended.

February 18, 2002. Carrie and I went to see, "A Beautiful Mind", the true story about mathematician and nobel prize winner Dr. John Nash, who battled with schizophrenia. Excellent movie. Then we went to Cheryl's birthday party. A fun afternoon and evening.

This morning I had to give myself a Zolodex implant because no one would give it to me. The medicentre was not familiar with it, my usual nurse, Henrietta, was not available, and the Cross says it's not part of their protocol. I actually did a good job!

February 19, 2002. Mom and I went to see Dr. JerrI Neilson, the lady who diagnosed herself with breast cancer when she was working in Antarctica. She was speaking at the Winspear tonight. Quite a funny lady, but she did not talk much about cancer!

February 20, 2002. Allison came over to pray this evening. It ends up that we have tea and then pray. I have to decide about radiation so we prayed for guidance. I got my bone scan and my chest X-ray results today and they are normal, so no metastases. I would like to see if this arimidex and UFT is going to work first but they want me to decide right away about radiation. I have to talk to Dr. Vazquez before I do anything. I do not like this "decide right away" business. I think my lifestyle changes will continue to make a big difference in the outcome.

February 21,2002. Met with Louise for supper after work. Dorothy, a native lady, shared her testimony at the Mars Hill meeting.

February 22, 2002. I'm fighting off a cold that I must have picked up from Soo, the student from Korea who is staying with me. It is a really bad one. I still went to work today but the cold totally wiped me out.

February 23, 2002. Went for a massage at one of the local spas but they refused to treat me because I have cancer. In their training schools here, they are taught that massage is contraindicated (not recommended) for cancer patients. That sure is different from the philosophy at Sanoviv. They teach that it helps boost the immune system. The therapist said if I bring in a doctor's order he will work on me, but until then he's afraid of being held liable for spreading the cancer. Good thing it is in Dr. Vazquez' orders. It was kinda frustrating.

Mim, Alan, Val, Cheryl, Monica and I went to see *Amalie*, nominated for best foreign picture. It was a fun evening.

Sunday, February 24, 2002. Got my income tax done today. Hope it comes back soon so I can pay off some of my medical expenses.

Psalm 30:2 really blessed me this morning: "O Lord my God, I called to you for help and you healed me."

Tuesday, February 26,2002. Henrietta, my alternative health nurse, examined me today after work. She's been on holidays for a month and before that I was in Sanoviv, so she had not seen me for 2 months. Henrietta thinks I've improved a lot in that time, and does not recommend jumping into radiation right away. I came away totally encouraged because she was so happy with my progress.

Wednesday, February 27, 2002. Visited with Allison. She's leaving for Ghana tomorrow, so it is our last prayer time for 6 weeks.

Thursday, February 28, 2002. Supper with Louise and Susan. Went to Lyle McWilliams' talk on *Fast Food Freddie*, how the corporate food culture is killing us softly. Learned about the number of reproductions a cell can go through before it dies. Something goes wacky with cancer cells and they keep reproducing.

Tuesday , March 5, 2002. Well it has been awhile. I visited with my cousin Janice on the weekend - had not seen her and François since Christmas Eve. Church was awesome. Visiting pastor, Wes Campbell taught about praying the scriptures, which reinforced what I have been doing. He said that our culture has lost the art of meditating. I agree with that. My church home group in the evening was pretty encouraging also.

Yesterday I took Mom to Max's Vegetarian restaurant. I think she was pretty happy I took her out. Afterwards, I went to my friend Verla's. Verla and I visited and prayed for awhile.

Finally I got my massage on Saturday. It was nothing like a Sanoviv massage. Oh well! Once you've had the best everything else is a let down. I wish all massage therapists could go down there for a few weeks and really learn a few things.

Thursday, March 7, 2002. Yesterday I spent some time on Dr. Lorraine Day's website. The website has new info. I reread Dr. Day's letter to cancer patients and she really stresses drinking 8 cups of carrot/apple juice a day, plus 4 cups of green juice. Wow have I got a long way to go! Today I managed three cups of carrot but I didn't start juicing until the afternoon. Since I have eight patients a day I will have to juice after every patient! I haven't even figured out how I'm going to do the green juice yet.

The weather is so unbelievably cold for this time of year - minus 25° Celsius with humidity. I have not been walking this week and the weight is no longer coming off. I surrender and get out the down-filled coat because the weather is not expected to warm up any time soon. Hard to believe it will officially be spring in two weeks.

Tonight, at Mars Hill, a Christian ministry, Cheryl taught about spending time in the desert before entering into the promised land. It is so true that God walks with us through the valley of the shadow of death.

Saturday, March 16, 2002. I did not look after myself as well as I should have this week. It was a bit too busy and exercise went out the window. Monday I had to call the plumber as my toilet was leaking, Tuesday I got together with Carrie to see *I Am Sam*, Wednesday was my University AlumnI dinner, and Thursday the plumber came back because the sink in the basement was dripping. Soo, a Korean student, is living down there. The bill stressed me out a bit, but I have been blessed that not much else has gone wrong with this house over the past seven years. Anyways, the end result of all this stress showed up in my colon hydrotherapy yesterday - hard pellets. Get more fibre girl!

Last night's television shows, *Air Farce* and *This Hour Has 22 Minutes* were hilarious. After them, I listened to my favourite doctor, Lorraine Day. I bought two more of her videos, *Sorting Through the Maze of Alternative Medicine* and *Believing is Seeing*. Her evaluation of different alternative therapies is very helpful. She speaks highly of colon therapy, massage, hydrotherapy, the Hallelujah Acres diet, and Ann Wigmore's diet. She does not specifically mention Oncolyn, AG-Immune, or any of the other supplements I have been taking, but she does say if it comes in a can or a bottle she doesn't want it. She says "You can't improve on God."

Tuesday, March 19, 2002. Woke up with an itchy welt on the side of my breast this morning. I didn't know if toxins were breaking through the skin or if something just irritated the skin. I decided to just carry on with God's plan and not worry about it. The welt was gone by the end of the day.

I went to Dina's for supper tonight. She wanted to borrow Dr. Day's video, so I took her *Believing is Seeing*.

Wednesday, March 20, 2002. Laurie hasn't mentioned her boyfriend for a long time, you say. Well I've been working through that one for months. He left the relationship in August last year. The timing was really bad for me, but I agree he had to have time by himself. Fortunately I have a fairly good network of friends, but I needed time to go through the grieving process and to regroup.

My room upstairs has become my sanctuary. I cannot hear Soo down in the basement at all so I feel it is just me and the Lord up here.

Friday, March 22, 2002. Had lunch with my friend Terry today. I had the lentil-nut loaf at Max's Vegetarian Restaurant. Awesome! Terry asked me where she could buy a juicer. She said that watching me go through this cancer ordeal is causing her to make changes in her diet.

I also picked up my MRI results at the Cross today. Good news! It has improved since the last one in November. That means my current program is working! I feel incredible joy. I watched the birds outside flying around and singing and I was flying with them! My friend Dina was so happy when I told her the good news. She wants to borrow all of Dr. Day's videos.

Sunday, March 24, 2002. Dr. Jesse Stoff was in Edmonton yesterday so I went to hear him. Dr. Stoff is the immunologist who developed the AG Immune product. He teaches that the immune system breaks down because of the PITTS. P is for poor nutrition, I is for infection, T is for toxins, the next T is for trauma and S is for stress. He confirmed that we should be eating organic, staying away from heavy metals, taking precautions when flying over 3500 ft (extra antioxidants), and having FUN!

Visualization: Cancer is Just a Bully

Monday, March 25, 2002. I have been thinking about the picture that God gave me while I was in Sanoviv. We did some work one evening visualizing our cancer disappearing. I saw that cancer is like a bully in a school yard, pushing other kids around and keeping the children in fear. But the principle of the school calls a meeting. In the meeting, the principle explains that the bully is just an insecure person who only has power because the other children allow the bully that power. Once the children stop giving this power to the bully, he can do no more harm. The children are given information and skills to use to stop the bully in his tracks. That is what cancer is like. It terrifies people because they don't understand it is an insecure cell that can only survive in an unhealthy environment. They need to be given skills to create a healthy environment.

Saturday, March 30, 2002. Since I live only a few blocks from the Cross cancer institute, I'm contemplating taking in ladies from out of town who need to come in for treatment. This idea came to me as I was relaxing and listening to God. I know I could be an encouragement to people as I've learned so much over the last year. Of course if the social worker in charge of the housing registry finds out I haven't followed all their treatment protocol, she may not even put me on the list! I'll phone on Monday and find out. Hopefully she won't even ask me if I'm a patient there.

Friday, April 5, 2002. I just got my first hair cut in a whole year! What a thrill! I have hair to cut! I went to a school of hairdressing so it did not cost much.

On Monday I had an appointment with the radiation oncologist. That brought me down emotionally for a couple of days. She "appeared" kind when she told me she would not order any more MRI's for me through the Cross, even though each successive one has shown steady improvement. This doesn't make any sense to me because it is one good way to tell if we're making progress with therapy. The doctors at the Cross liked it as a marker when I was taking their chemo, but now that I'm taking an alternative treatment they say an MRI is not a good marker. She had me doubting my choice of therapy to the extent that I didn't do any juicing on Tuesday. I had supper with my old friend Barb and her husband Paul on that day and Barb encouraged me that it just takes longer to heal when you are fighting it the natural way. It is easier to slash and burn.

On Wednesday I had my Vega treatment after work. My tumor responded very well to the audiocolour. I have noticed many times that my breast has been much softer afterward. Henrietta encouraged me that we could find another way to get an MRI done in a couple of months. She also said that this lack of cooperation of the cancer institute is common with most cancer patients she sees who chose to take control of their own therapy. The oncologist also told me that she would do more tests if I decided to have radiation, to make sure nothing has spread, but otherwise no tests. She seemed really kind when she was telling me that, but in reality it is a way to strong-arm someone - do it our way or we will not help you. I am welcome to go and talk to her if I need to but I do not know how productive that would be.

Tuesday, April 16, 2002. The PapimI machine arrived in Edmonton over a week ago and life has not been the same since. I go every evening and weekends for treatments so there is not much free time to write. The PapimI was developed by a Dr. Pappas from Greece who has a PhD in Physics. He was doing research on lightening bolts in the States with a colleague who had terminal cancer. The colleague unexpectedly was cured by being in that work environment. This discovery led Dr. Pappas to redirect his research focus towards developing a biomedical device that would cure cancer. My understanding is that an increase of negative ions exists in the air after an electrical storm and that these ions are necessary for good health. The PapimI creates negative ions, making our bodies more alkaline. Cancer does not survive in an alkaline environment. That I know from Sanoviv.

Then Monday I was scared to death because my tumor seemed to get harder. I thought I was getting worse so the PapimI tech, Debbie, called the Biomedical PhD in California and we described the situation to him. What he said made me so happy I almost jumped out of my skin. Obviously he had years of experience because he knew right away what was going on. He told me that when the body realizes it has a chance to actually kill this tumor, it encapsulates it, and cuts off its blood supply. The hardness can last for a few days to a week and then it gets really soft. That is exactly what happened - by the next day the breast felt normal.

Wednesday, April 24, 2002. I am still on a steep learning curve but I haven't had much time to write about it because everyday after work I have been going for papimI treatments. My joints are so much better since I started that I have not had to take any Vioxx. It has been almost 3 weeks now. The papimI has been allowed into North America on the basis that it helps to alleviate pain. Research studies on pain management have been started in the States and now in Canada. People with PapimI machines are not authorized to do studies on cancer here. However a study was recently completed in Germany on 60 women with stage one breast cancer and all 60 cancer patients had a complete recovery. This study will be submitted to a scientific journal for publication, which I hope will not take too long. I understand it can take up to six months. I have been getting exhausted going every day so we're going to cut back the treatments to twice a week to give my body time to recuperate in between. The telephone support person in California said I am going through a healing crisis and my liver and lymph system need time to process after so many treatments. I do feel nervous sometimes because this is all new territory.

Wednesday, May 1, 2002. The jury is still out on the PapimI machine - good or bad? I phoned Sanoviv to get their opinion because I know that they had considered buying it. Dr. Peña called and I described to him all that I am experiencing - pain in the breast with some inflammation and a seeming enlargement of the tumor. He told me that another clinic down in Mexico is getting good results with it and that all reports so far have been positive. As for the inflammation, he thought it could be a good thing as it usually means something unwanted is being attacked. Of course it is difficult to say for sure over the telephone, without a physical exam, but he knows how cancer usually behaves. He suggested continuing for one more week so I am considering it.

Meanwhile, spiritually I need to stay grounded. Terry, a new lady at church, and Allison came and prayed with me on Monday. It really strikes me that the people who are the most broken are the ones who reach out to others. Many in our church are so content that it does not occur to them to reach out, but Terry, who just got baptised, and who is going through trials, is the one who comes. I felt Jesus' compassion through her and through Allison.

Jesus feels very close right now. After work, I just wanted to come home and be alone with Him. Psalm 41:1 really struck me: "Blessed is he who has regard for the weak; the Lord delivers him in times of trouble." I believe that the Lord is delivering me in my time of trouble. I got out my guitar and worshipped Him and felt His presence in the room.

Friday, May 3, 2002. So much for Comedy Night on CBC (Canadian Broadcasting) - the hockey game was on. I got some painting and cleaning done instead, so I guess it was for the best.

Today I had a patient who was complaining about a breast lump and the doctors are not taking her seriously. I told her my story and then she did not feel as frustrated anymore because somebody finally believed her. They are telling her she is stressed out and is imagining everything. Yes stress does do things to the body, but at the same time, a woman knows her own breast and should be listened to. Not being believed can be stressful too. She was from Europe and was very open to natural healing and prevention. I gave her a list of resources. I thought it was odd that a woman with breast pain would be sent for nerve conduction tests, but God works all things together for good!

Saturday, May 4, 2002. George Malkmus' book, "God's Way to Ultimate Health" arrived at the bookstore, finally![16] I ordered it two months ago but the publisher ran out of copies and it had to be sourced from another distributor. I cannot put it down. His testimony is amazing! He was diagnosed with colon cancer in 1974, and because his mother had just died of colon cancer after having chemo, surgery and radiation, he did not want to go those routes. Instead, he went on the Gerson plan and his cancer cleared up within a year, along with several other of his physical problems! The Gerson plan is basically a vegan diet with lots of juicing and it has been instrumental in helping many people with cancer. This led Dr. Malkmus to develop the Hallelujah Acres Ministry, which has helped many thousands of people over the years. The scientific explanations in his book, which was co-written by Micheal Dye, are very clear, and the biblical exposition is excellent. Who better to do a biblical exposition than a Baptist pastor, which is what Rev. Malkmus is.

In my visualization, the principal of the school gave information to the students so they would be able to create a healthy environment. A bully cannot function in a place where he has no support. The principal of this school is God and He is teaching me step by step how to make my body into an environment where cancer, the bully, cannot survive.

Beginning to See the End of the Tunnel

Tuesday, May 7, 2002. Today I can hardly contain myself! I saw my oncologist and he could not feel or see any difference between my two breasts. He said that what I have done obviously worked and he looked genuinely happy for me. I told him, his nurse and his resident that I was following Dr. Lorraine Day's plan and they all asked who is Dr. Lorraine Day, and what is her plan? I told them they would just have to get her video because I could not do her plan justice in five minutes. I also said if they put their patients on this plan they'd all be walking out of the hospital. They seemed to think that would be an OK idea. Maybe they would like to help more people than they actually do.

I think Mexican clinics just went up in my doctors estimation, because five months ago he thought they were crazy for putting me on Zoladex and Arimidex; now he is saying he will prescribe Arimidex for me, because it obviously worked. However, I would still have to pay for it because it is usually only given to metastatic patients. My big question at the moment is, now that I'm on a completely vegan diet, getting at least a couple of cups of carrot juice, daily walks of about 40 minutes, and all the rest of the plan, do I need to continue taking estrogen blockers (Arimidex and Zoladex)? I don't consume the animal products that are full of hormones and fat anymore - I have not even had salmon since before Christmas. If I have to, I will take the drugs, but they cost me over ten thousand dollars per year.

Friday, May 10, 2002. Reading George Malkmus' book reveals to me a whole new world. There are many people who have been healed of degenerative diseases by changing their diet and lifestyle. It appears to me there is more than enough scientific evidence that lifestyle changes can heal disease. I keep hearing the medical community saying that changing the diet is not enough to combat cancer, but I don't think it has been seriously studied. Why study carrot juice when so much money can be made by the pharmaceutical companies selling drugs? Pharmaceutical companies are always announcing the newest and latest drug. Who cares about the lowly carrot? I think God cares about it - He created it!

It is also amazing to me that George Malkmus' book is not on every pastors' bookshelf. The first book he wrote, *Why Christians get Sick* is not even stocked at the local bookstore. How many pastors pray for their people with cancer and they still die? Is time even spent at church teaching us how to keep our bodies as a temple for God? Certainly no one has given me Dr. Malkmus' book since I was diagnosed, leading me to assume the pastors don't have it, or if they do, they don't understand its importance.

Sunday, May 12, 2002. What a beautiful mother's day! The sun was shining and the sky was blue. Jennifer, Hugh, mom, two of Jenn's kids, her mom-in-law and I went for supper on Whyte Avenue. I got my mom a gift certificate for Planet Organic, a natural food health store that I shop at frequently. She's making a few lifestyle changes!

There is a very interesting quote in George Malkmus' book: "It is my view that the vegetarian manner of living, by its purely physical effect on the human temperament, would most beneficially influence the lot of mankind." - Albert Einstein,1940. Wow! A real genius thinks it is a good idea. Another quote by an evangelist named Lester Roloff got my attention: "The secret of a live, clean body is live, clean food - fresh vegetables, juices, fruit, and nice green salads...I do not live completely without a cook stove, but because of its overuse, it has become the murderer of the human race." Lester Roloff is the person who encouraged George Malkmus to go the raw food route, and when he did his tumor went away. It seems to me like it should be standard treatment protocol for anyone with cancer. It's like a hidden treasure that you have to go seeking for. I wonder who's trying to keep it a secret? Wouldn't it be nice if we had Organic Salad Express all over the country, instead of Fast Food Freddie?

Wednesday, May 22, 2002. I feel really tired. Monday was a holiday so Teresa and Jared and I went for a 2-hour walk to Hawelak Park and back. I also mowed the lawn and planted some lettuce, so I guess I have a reason to be tired. I do wonder if the cancer is still there, however.

Dr. Tal brought me some Barley Green to work today. George Malkmus and Lorraine Day both said it is crucial to the healing process. Barley Green is the juice of the young barley plant, which is dried in a process that preserves the vitamins, minerals and enzymes. Dr. Yoshihide Hagiwara, a Japanese research pharmacologist spent years developing this product. He reflects on the vitality of the green leaf in his book *Green Barley Essence*: "I cannot but feel that man has overlooked the power of green in favour of science and technology and modern rationalism." I say amen to that. Barley Green is not quite as strong as wheatgrass so it is a bit easier to get down when mixed with some fresh juice. Mrs. Tal has been taking Barley Green for years so I bought some from her. I definitely will continue to take it.

Friday, May 24, 2002. Went to the oxygen bar after work. The owner said he had been concerned about me 'cause he had not seen me for awhile. I try to get there as often as I can because I know cancer can't live in a highly oxygenated environment. Scientists have found that the oxygen content of our air is greatly depleted from what it was years ago and humans are in an oxygen crisis right now. I know now that for cancer to grow in my body, my internal oxygen levels had to be very low. Fresh juices have a high water content and water is made of oxygen, so when I was not juicing and eating fresh vegetables I was not getting enough oxygen. Coffee, sugar and all the other junk I used to consume require huge amounts of oxygen for metabolism. That does not leave enough for all the other needs the body has. No wonder I was so challenged whenever I did anything aerobic. I was given oxygen treatment everyday when I was at Sanoviv and I can't understand why it is not given to cancer patients at the Cross. It is apparently a known fact that radiation kills more cancer cells when the person's body is highly oxygenated, so why is oxygen not given to patients?

Wednesday, May 29, 2002. It is really exiting how many people are getting into juicing. One of the fellows in my prayer group at church wanted to help me and I told him I needed help with juicing because juicing eight cups of carrot juice a day gets really tedious. After I showed Stewart how to make the juice and he tasted how good it was, he really got into it. Now Stewart comes every day that I work and makes a few glasses of juice for me and some for himself. When I told him it helps curb the appetite for sweet junk food, he was really impacted. I am very happy that this is blessing him because he is a huge blessing to me. Another lady in the same group who lives right on my way to work offered to make me a cup in the morning. Each morning as I make my way to work, I stop in at her house for a short time, then I carry on to work. JudI is a neat lady - she and her husband have been vegetarian for years, and their little daughter has never been in a MacDonald's. What an example!

I made a decision to go back on Arimidex and Zoladex. Dr. Vazquez was quite emphatic about it, and he has not let me down yet, so I am going to trust him. I will be on them for another three months. At that time Dr. Vazquez and I will revisit and decide. The Arimidex costs almost $200/mo. and the Zoladex is $500/mo., neither of which is covered by the provincial health care plan. That just gets added to my $50,000 credit line. I keep telling myself that I invested more in my house and I'm worth more than my house, but really the treatment I received at Sanoviv should be available here for everyone. A lot more lives would be saved, and there would be fewer recurrences, because people would learn the skills they need to stay well.

Take sprouting for example. The sprouting class we had in Sanoviv was excellent. The instructors gave us charts showing how long it takes for each type of seed, bean or nut to sprout, the number of daily rinses to give them, and how long their sprouts grow. The teachers explained to us that sprouts contain large amounts of enzymes necessary for digestion. When we eat cooked food all the time we are not getting the needed enzymes because cooking kills them. The body then is forced to use up its finite supply of enzymes in order to digest all the dead food we eat, leaving us in a negative situation. Now I have two sprouting jars and hope to get more so I can have fresh sprouts on all my salads. The ideal diet is at least 85 per cent raw, and that is my eventual goal, but I am making the change slowly.

Thursday, Jun 6, 2002. I discovered Dr. Norman Walker's book, *Fresh Vegetable and Fruit Juices*.[17] In my readings I kept coming across references to this man who lived to be 118 years old. Dr. Walker made such a huge contribution to the science of raw food nutrition and juicing. In this new vegan culture I live in, Dr. Walker is a shining example to all. Norman Walker explains what is in each of the vegetable juices and they sound so good I want to go out and fill my fridge with spinach, asparagus, Jerusalem artichokes, and celery to add them to the carrot juice. He recommends straight carrot juice and five oz of carrot juice mixed with three oz of spinach for cancer patients. A total of eight cups or more of these juices per day is good. Right now I am mixing Barley Green with carrot/apple juice, but I'll try spinach in one or two cups. Dr. Walker says it does not matter if you like the taste, when your health is compromised you do not have a choice. I did not know that spinach contains oxalic acid, which is useful for helping to clean out the intestines. If the spinach is raw, the oxalic acid works, but if it is cooked, it becomes inorganic and can form oxalic acid crystals in the kidneys, causing pain. Unfortunately, I love cooked spinach and will have to develop a liking for the raw form.

Fortunately, I love carrot juice. Dr. Walker says that: "Carrot juice is composed of a combination of elements, which nourish the entire system, helping to normalize its weight as well as its chemical balance." (p 30) Also: "If properly extracted from fresh, clean, good quality raw carrots, carrot juice is very rich in the vital organic alkaline elements sodium and potassium." (p28) When he says properly extracted, he is referring to the method of triturating (pulverizing) the vegetable and then squeezing the pulp through a hydraulic press. This is what the Norwalk juicer does. I am now finding out that this high quality juicer that I keep hearing about is his namesake.

Sunday, June 9, 2002. Today Teresa and I made carrot/spinach juice. I was amazed at how mild the spinach juice tasted. I thought it would be strong and hard to get down.

Saturday, June 15, 2002. I'm in the midst of reading yet another success story from the world of natural medicine - the Jason Winters Story. I was going to go to bed early Friday night, but I started reading the book... it is now 1:00 a.m.! I relate to so many aspects of his struggle, especially his faith and hope.

After a sleep and a trip to the farmer's market, I finished *A Prescription For Life, The Jason Winter's story*.[18] Jason Winters was diagnosed with infiltrating squamous cell carcinoma in 1977 at the age of 46, the same age I was when I was diagnosed. He underwent radiation and then he was supposed to have his tongue, jaw bone, neck muscles and the inside of his throat removed. To that Jason said an emphatic "no" and began searching the world to find a better way to deal with his problem. Jason's first visit was to Mexico where he was given laetrile, which helped him for a time, but ultimately did not solve the problem. He also made some diet changes at that time.

Then Jason Winters began to search the Bible and other religious books. He found that often herbs were mentioned for healing. Through his research, he came to the belief that herbalene was the most powerful of the ancient healing herbs for tumors. Jason found out that it grows only in Asia and was available in Singapore.

Using credit, which again I relate to, Jason flew to Singapore and found a lady who sold him some of the herb. She made a liquid concentrate from the roots of the herb by boiling them for hours. The tea did not shrink his tumor but it did prevent it from growing. This herb may also be known by another name as well as herbalene.

The next herb Jason Winters tried was chaparral, which comes from the creosote bush, prevalent in Arizona. He remembered that the Indians used to drink this tea when he was on the set of a western movie in his earlier years. So Jason went to Arizona to obtain some chaparral. The tea was bitter. It also did not shrink his tumor but it did prevent the tumor from growing, so Jason kept taking it.

The third trip Jason Winters made was to England where the use of herbs was more accepted in medical practice. In England, Jason was introduced to red clover, which he also began to take in tea form. He brewed all these teas separately and then one day, in pain and desperation he got the inspiration to brew them together. It was then that his tumor began to shrink. He drank a gallon of it everyday and within nine weeks his tumor was gone! This was the birth of the Jason Winters formula, which is currently sold around the world.

It is Jason's mission that I most relate to. Jason wants to see health care focus on prevention rather than treatment, and he wants to see the orthodox and unorthodox practitioners work together. This has been my dream for years and now it has become a passion. Interestingly, it is also a conviction of Prince Charles. Prince Charles writes the following about the Foundation for Integrated Medicine in London: "I am convinced that the integration of complementary and orthodox medical practices is urgently needed. It is all about breaking down artificial barriers of geography, culture and education so that we can bring the sum of human knowledge and experience to bear in caring even better for those who suffer from ill health or disability." (p158, *A Prescription For Life*)

There is one scripture that all of my mentors have quoted. Dr. Lorraine Day, George Malkmus, Dr. Don Colbert, Sir Jason Winters, and Dr. Norman Walker all quote Genesis 1:29: "Behold, I have given you the seed-bearing plants throughout the earth and all the fruit trees for your food." I believe this to be the scriptural basis for a vegan diet, which I am thriving on. The Genesis 1:29 Diet!

Sunday, June 23, 2002. I have another book to add to my growing book review: *Your Body's Many Cries For Water* by F. Batmanghelidj, affectionately known as Dr. Batman by those who know him.[19] This book has in-depth medical explanations. It is amazing how many signs our body gives us that it is thirsty. When we get dehydrated, our body releases a lot of histamine, which causes allergic reactions. It makes me wonder if that is why I had allergies when I was younger because I do not think I drank much water. Dehydration can also contribute to disc degeneration, high blood pressure, diabetes, depression, and other problems. Dr. "Batman" is calling for an overhaul of the medical paradigm, which currently treats these problems with medication without trying to rehydrate the person first. I have started asking people who suffer from these problems if they drink 8-10 glasses of water a day and none of them do!

Tuesday, June 25, 2002. I've been pruning many dead branches on the trees in my yard over the last couple of days. It occurred to me that I never wanted to prune my trees before I got sick, but now that I see the results from getting rid of bad habits (dead wood), I want to prune everything in sight!

Also I meditated on Psalm 118:17 today: "I will not die but live, and will proclaim what the Lord has done." Yes!

Saturday, June 29, 2002. George Malkmus' book, *Why Christians get Sick* arrived by special order at the Christian book store this week. It is amazing to me that they do not carry it on a regular basis considering all of the Christians who are sick these days.

This book was first published in 1989, but I have been in Christian circles for 26 years and never heard this teaching until I started listening to Lorraine Day M.D. There seems to be great resistance to healthy eating in the church.[20] People get prayed for yet they remain sick because nobody is teaching them to change the way they eat. It is easy to take the wide road that the rest of the world is taking instead of walking down the narrow road that God calls us to. This sounds harsh I realize, but gluttony is just as serious as drunkenness or any of the other vices listed in the Bible. I know because I had to learn the hard way what it does to you. I am not saying that prayer is not important, rather I am saying that we need to do our part. There are too many sticky, sugary desserts at church functions!

Dr. Malkmus mentions that Seventh Day Adventists, as a group, live six years longer than the average American. They have included teaching on how to take care of the body in their doctrine:

meat, coffee and tea are not recommended. Ellen G. White, the founder of the Seventh Day Adventists, has written extensively on health issues. I have ordered one of her books because she is highly recommended by Dr. Lorraine Day. I can remember at Pentecostal gatherings, making fun of Seventh Day Adventists because they were missing out on the joys of coffee drinking, and what damage could coffee possibly do? Well the joke is really on us because caffeine increases blood pressure and damages the liver and kidneys - slowly, so you do not notice it until it is too late. It's like the proverbial frog in the pot of water - if you heat the water slowly the frog will not jump out, but if you put the frog in a boiling pot it will jump out right away. I remember taking my first sip of coffee at age fifteen and wanting to spit it out. That should have been warning enough for me!

Sunday, June 30, 2002. I very much would like to be part of *Back to the Garden Health Ministries*. It's an informational ministry that George Malkmus began at Hallelujah Acres. Training is offered several times a year. I may not be able to make it this year because I do not think that travelling is a good idea yet, and neither do the doctors at Sanoviv. My reason for writing this book is so others can benefit from my struggle. It has taken me a year and a half so far to assemble all this information and I know there is still more to learn.

Meanwhile I'm helping to promote Dr. Lanzagorta's lecture. He is the medical outreach doctor from Sanoviv and he will be speaking here in Edmonton on July 21, 2002. I already have several friends coming because they have seen what Sanoviv did for me. The lecture is titled: *The Price We Pay for Living in a Modern World, and the Way Out*. Over a thousand people are expected to attend.

Monday, July 1, Canada Day, 2002. My friend JudI suggested I put everything that is in plastic bags into glass jars so I started doing that today. I have heard before that plastic can leach into the food and it has estrogen-like components that are carcinogenic. Things actually look better in glass jars anyway. JudI told me that the guy who invented plastic is now sorry that he did, but it is so entrenched in our society that it is hard to escape from. Plastic is something I have to do more research on. Off to a Canada Day picnic!

Friday, July 5, 2002. This week has just flown by. Henrietta tested me on the Vega Test Expert machine on Tuesday. My carcinoma reading has improved from three weeks ago. In fact it is zero! My highest readings were from my liver and my joints but even they improved. Because I still believe machines can make mistakes, I asked her to manually check the breast and she said there was no tumor to be felt. I have gained a tremendous trust in her over this past year and I feel really happy when she says it seems normal!

At the health store I found a book, which I am surprised is not on the headline news every night. It's called: *You* ***Can*** *Prevent Breast Cancer!* by Harvey Diamond, the author of *Fit For Life*. Every once in awhile there is some news about a new "break-through" drug treatment, which causes people to think that should they ever have the misfortune of developing cancer; there are better ways of treating it. What this leads people to think is that there is no way of preventing it in the first place, and if they do get it the only way to treat it is with drugs. Wrong! This book came out in 1995, it gives clear evidence that cancer can be prevented, but the majority of people do not know because they've never heard.[21] Why? Everybody knows about what happened Sept 11, 2001, because it was plastered all over the news for days and weeks and months. We still hear about it and this affects us when we travel. Do we do anything about the terrorist fast food industry that is killing millions of people? No! What about the dairy industry?

I have been doing a lot of thinking about what I would have done if my cancer had been detected earlier. The first part of my book focuses on the problems I had with misdiagnoses. Now that I know cancer can be prevented by following God's Health Plan, I would have gone on the plan immediately to prevent the cancer from progressing to stage three. Whether the lump showed on the mammogram or not, no lump is normal, so a person needs to do a major detox to get rid of it. There is so much talk about the importance of early detection, but very little talk about how not to get cancer in the first place. Yes there is lip service paid to "healthy living" by the medical profession but no doctor told me that healthy living included going off milk products, sugar, caffeine, and meat. I was not told to get my colon cleansed or to jump on a minI trampoline to keep my lymph system healthy. To this day they harass me for drinking fresh carrot juice. It amazes me that they tell women, "you have to have your breast cut off" and women go and do it. Why don't they tell women, "you have to go to a detox spa for a month and get cleaned out"? It would probably cost the health care system less than a mastectomy in the long run, when you think of all the complications after a surgery like that. And surgery doesn't solve the problem because it doesn't deal with the lifestyle factors that contributed to it in the first place. Even as this day passes another woman has had her breast removed and still lives with the fear that "it" (the bully) could come back.

Harvey Diamond, in *You **Can** Prevent Breast Cancer* talks about a huge study that was done in China, definitively linking diet to health, which was inaugurated in 1983. It is called The Cornell Oxford China Project on Nutrition, Health and Environment, or the China Health Project for short. The coordinator of the project was Dr. T. Colin Campbell, a nutritional biochemist at Cornell University (p136). It was found that the Chinese obtain 7 per cent of their protein from animal products, whereas Americans obtain 70 per cent of their protein from animal products (p137). Dr. Campbell found: "In those few regions in China where meat and dairy consumption has begun to increase - notably the heavily westernized cities - it has been closely followed by a higher incidence of cancer, heart disease and diabetes. Once these people start eating more animal products, that is when all the mischief starts." (p142) All this is relevant to women because the death rate from breast cancer is **five** times higher for Americans than it is for the Chinese. The first seven years of data from this project were released in the mid-1990's. How many North American women have heard of it? Why is it not on the news? Would advertising money from the milk producers have anything to do with it?

Wednesday, July 10, 2002. Just this week the cover feature of Time magazine was on vegetarianism, and how more and more Americans are converting. I was just saying that we need more news coverage of the benefits of vegetarianism and presto; there it was plastered on the front of *Time Magazine*.

Sunday, July 14, 2002. It has been impossible to write for the last few days because it has been 34° Celcius! These kind of record-breaking temperatures leave everybody feeling very listless. Every time I tried to come upstairs to write I felt this massive wall of heat pushing me back downstairs.

Healing the Wounds

Go to Him

I came to talk to you one day
You always seemed so far away
I wanted to know where you were at
I never thought that you would do that

After that time the world became black
My mind and spirit were way off track
Nobody knew why I went crazy
Why on earth I became so lazy

The wall around me grew really thick
Just leave her alone she's really sick
How could I explain why I went wild?
I didn't know, I was just a child

In this world of darkness I was all alone
No one could read my face of stone
Then one day someone saw my plight
She told me about a kingdom of light

The King of this world will care for you
If you go to Him, He'll make you anew
Your mind and spirit will start to clear
Go to Him, it's safe to draw near

He doesn't Lord it over others
He walks with those who love their brothers
My wasted life he made anew
What He did for me, He can do for you

I sing His songs, I know His grace
Now people see joy upon my face
I feel His love every single day
His spirit is with me, His word lights my way

Oh man in darkness, Oh man in pride
Can you open your heart and let Him inside?
He knows where you're at, He sees your plight
Can you leave the darkness and walk in the light?

I agree with Dr. Lorraine Day that a person needs to come to a place of forgiveness when wrong things are done to you. It took me a long time to come to that place. It may not be possible to ever change the behavior of another person, but it is possible to forgive. In order to heal, it is crucial to forgive.

For that reason, I believe it to be wise not to write in detail about this incident. I can say that I became so depressed I was taken to see a psychiatrist. The real cause was not mentioned, and the doctor sure did not pick up the signs. Not many people talked about it in those days. It was 1968. I left home when I was 17 and did one semester of University. I could not concentrate so I went wandering the world at the age of 18. I lived on a kibbutz in Israel for several months. When I came home things were unbearable. I was put in the hospital for awhile. Over the next several years, my father left for long periods of time. In 1988 he married one of his grad students. His mind was anywhere but on being emotionally close to his children.

I became one of the hippies who rebelled against materialism because I did not see material things producing much relationship between people. Then in 1976 I gave my heart to Jesus. Everybody thought that was going to be another phase, but Jesus is always there. I will never leave Him. He gave me life and hope and dignity. Unfortunately I was too shy around men. Marriages were taking place on a regular basis at my church but I was always passed by. I was so nervous, I could hardly carry on a conversation. My father's uncontrolled temper deeply affected my self-esteem. But slowly my mind started to heal, as I focused my mind on God, and I was able to finish my training as an EEG tech and begin a stable career. I learned to stand up for myself.

I wrote the above poem when I was working through facing the reality of what happened to me as a young person. I was 39 before I started to talk openly about it. I only include it here to say that I carried a lot of pain for many years. This kind of pain can kill you if you do not deal with it. I had to grieve and move on. It has not yet been possible to resolve the issue yet, but I have faith that it will be. The pain that you feel when you realize that you could die and a significant person would not come to see you is indescribable. I asked God to meet my needs in this area and I decided to live. There were many times in the past that I wanted to die and I am sure my mind was giving that message to my body. Before I went to Sanoviv, I did not realize how powerful the mind-body connection was. I do not want to dwell on what I do not have however, cause that will just make me sick. I just have to be aware of what happened so that it does not affect my relationships with other people.

As a young person, that pain drove me to the One who shed his blood for us. I felt so much empathy for other people who were suffering. It was so evident to me that we had so much in North America as far as Bibles and food and opportunities for education. All I lived for was to go on missions to the poorest countries in the world, to help alleviate suffering for a few people. My vacations were spent on mission trips and I loved it, but I was not looking after myself. I did not feel at liberty to even laugh much when there was so much suffering in the world. After getting cancer, I learned that laughter is part of the healing process and if I want to live I better learn to laugh.

Thursday, July 18, 2002. Dr. Lanzagorta will be in Edmonton on Sunday to talk about Sanoviv. I was asked to do a 10-minute testimony part way through his lecture, which I am really happy to do. There are so many people who need hope and information. You cannot have faith if it's not based on truth. So far I have six guests coming for the afternoon session and eight for the evening but I think more will be buying tickets at the door. It will be so nice to have Henrietta, Allison, JudI and the many others who have stood by me during this trial attending the meeting.

Wednesday, July 24, 2002. It has been a couple of weeks since I stopped taking anti-depressants. Usually after a week I am a basket case, crying and very tired. Now I am waking up naturally when the sun comes up which today was around 5 a.m. I cleaned a window, watered the garden, did my rebounding, made a flower arrangement, and now I'm going in to work! I think Dr. Lorraine Day is right that fresh air, exercise, sunlight and eating vegan does help heal depression. I've tried to go off before but have never been able to last this long. Praise God!

Allison videotaped my testimony at Dr. Lanzagorta's lecture on Sunday. At the second session, one man told me he came back with his wife because he was so impressed with my story in the afternoon. I am pleased that God used me to touch someone. I shared what I had learned about the connection between milk and breast cancer from Dr. Jane Plant, which was confirmed when I got to Sanoviv. The difference in treatment approaches was my main point. Dr. Lanzagorta's lecture was truly amazing. You are in awe of God when you listen to him. He gave a new meaning to what a good grandma is - it is not someone who bakes, gives goodies to the kids and weighs 250 pounds. That is not love. That is sending yourself and your loved ones to an early grave.

Dr. Lanzagorta's PowerPoint presentation was indeed powerful. He used the analogy of a smoke alarm going off in one room, so the person calls the fire department and they come and shut off the alarm, not doing anything about the fire. Then the alarm goes off in another room and the fire department comes and unhooks it. This continues until the whole house is on fire and the person loses his house. This is exactly what happens to people when they go to the doctor - they get a pill, which puts out the body's alarm for awhile but does not deal with the problem. In the case of cancer they cut out the piece of cancer but the medical profession does not deal with the factors causing the cancer in the first place.

Friday, July 26, 2002. For the next two weeks I am off because Dr. Tal is on holidays. Yeah! I am looking forward to writing, reading, relaxing, getting together with friends and trying out some new recipes. Today I did dry skin brushing. At Sanoviv they gave us each a dry skin brush to take home. They taught us that lightly brushing the skin stimulates the lymphatic system, which is just under the surface of the skin. You always brush towards the centre of your body to promote drainage of the lymphatic fluid. I also did rebounding, which stimulates the lymphatic system as well.

The other day I came across an oncology bulletin titled: *Why do doctors delay in diagnosing breast cancer?* They were quoting from the Archives of Internal Medicine, June 24/02: "Some physicians hold back on their suspicions of a woman having a breast tumor and this delay can affect survival." (162:1343-1348, 2002) Boy do I know that from experience. One of the doctors who misdiagnosed me actually told me that she did not like telling people they had cancer, because she would rather give them good news than bad. Well isn't that sweet? Most people would rather know the truth sooner than later. Better yet, they would rather be told how to prevent the cancer in the first place.

Saturday, July 27, 2002. I have been experiencing terrible joint pain, which I know is a side-effect of the Zoladex. The pain been really slowing me down, but I remembered that Dr. Walker had said that grapefruit is good for arthritis, so I had one this morning and it does feel much better.

Sometimes I forget the seriousness of what I am dealing with and I eat out too much. Even though I'm always eating vegetarian, much of the food is cooked, and devitalized. My biggest challenge is eating the majority of my food raw. Last Saturday, a bunch of us went to a restaurant, which serves mock meat, made out of tofu, soya bean, wheat gluten and wheat protein. Well, I do not think that is a good idea to do again - the muscles in the bowel are not powerful enough to move "glue" along the way. If I did not get colon therapy I do not know when those sticky clumps would have come out. Gluten = Glue.

I found a good quote today that accurately describes what I am going through. "It may be hard to follow this diet, as the cancer seems to crave the dead, demineralized foods the same as a smoker craves tobacco, but do not give in - you must starve the cancer cells while building up good healthy cells, and the craving will grow less and less as time goes by." (p97, *Make Your Juicer Your Drug Store*)[22] Anybody changing to a raw food diet could relate to that. I remember one of the companions of a patient at Sanoviv left for a day so he could go and get some cooked food!

Tuesday, July 30, 2002. The last few days have been an adventure. On Sunday Teresa and her son Jared and I went saskatoon-berry picking. We found a huge patch in the Edmonton river valley and we each got a bag full of the berries. There are so many that

Allison and I went again the next day and got a bunch more. This may not sound exciting but when one is living on organic fruits and vegetables, to find bags of free fruit is a God-send. I am taking my neighbour Alma tomorrow afternoon to pick some more.

Yesterday I finally found the books by Ellen G. White that I've been looking for. Dr. Lorraine Day had recommended her books but I haven't been able to find them in any of the regular bookstores. One of my health books mentioned that Ellen White is the main founder of the Seventh Day Adventist Church so I was able to locate her material at one of their book mobiles. Her *Ministry of Healing* seems like another hidden gem. It was written about 100 years ago but the principles are still as true today as they were then. She emphasizes the need for fresh air and sunlight, which many people don't get any more.[23]

Thursday, August 1, 2002. Reading John Robbin's book *Diet For A New World* stirs up so much in my heart. He has a cartoon inside that says it all. It is a man with a belly so huge he cannot see his own feet. Under his belly, are three starving orphans sitting around an empty bowl. Not only do we have a lot of food in North America, we eat too much of the wrong food. He has a lot of documentation that shows how much grain it takes to feed cattle. If all the land that is taken up to feed beef were used to feed people, more would be fed.[24] John Robbins is the son of the owner the Baskin- Robbins ice cream chain, and when he learned how much damage dairy did to people he refused to take over the family business.

Sunday, August 4, 2002. Had some friends over for a pot luck on Friday evening. One of the most common questions I get asked is "where do you get your protein?" I used to think that protein came only from meat and dairy products and that vegans were protein deficient but I am finding more and more information to the contrary: "Most people seem to think protein needs to come from meat and dairy products. Even those more "in the know" about alternative health subscribed for a long time to the theory that vegetable proteins were somehow second-class and required proper "combining" to be complete. But vegetables carry all the amino acids (the building blocks of protein) the body needs. Not every vegetable has every one, of course, but if you are eating a wide variety of vegetables, especially dark green and dark green leafy vegetable, and supplementing with grasses, you are getting plenty of all the essential amino acids."[25] (p61, The pH Miracle) Now I can confidently tell people that the average North American gets over 100 grams of protein per day and we only need about 40 grams.

The other question people ask me is 'where do you get your calcium?' I am finding out that the biggest cause of osteoporosis is not lack of calcium but excess protein leaching calcium into the urine. It is actually a well-documented phenomenon called protein-induced hypercalciuria.[26] So as long as I am eating lots of different vegetables I am covered, and the calcium that I do have will not be leached out. I do take a Usana vitamin supplement that has calcium citrate in it as well. All the time that I was eating meat, I was peeing out calcium! Those restaurant deals where they give you a half chicken are not a good plan!

Tuesday, August 6, 2002. Yesterday Teresa, Jared and I went raspberry picking. O Heaven! My favorite fruit. It looked like it was going to be a rainy holiday Monday but the sun came through. We each got about a bucket full. I wanted to fill the freezer with berries. I don't think I will get quite that much but I am really thankful for all the free fruit God has provided. I like fruit more than vegetables so I have to be careful not to eat too much fruit and leave out the vegetables! Fruit has more sugar than vegetables do.

Today I saw a doctor who specializes in nutritional medicine. He checked my blood pressure and it is now down to 115/75! Before this diet change a year ago it was around 140/90! More confirmation I'm on the right track!

Friday, August 9, 2002. What a scary day. I got my progress notes from the Cross yesterday and my doctor's final conclusion was that because I have refused surgery and radiation I "would not be curable." I went to sleep with those words in my head and I woke up in a state of fear and panic. Words are so powerful.

They can bring life or death to a person. The word "incurable" should not be used because it produces fear. By the time I got to my vega appointment, I was hyperventilating and crying. Henrietta was able to calm me down somewhat. When I got to colon hydrotherapy, Sharon was concerned and was able to reassure me some more. Sometimes everything gets overwhelming. I have been wanting to get another ultrasound and scan done so I know we are on the right track with the therapy that I have chosen but they will not give me one because I am not going for radiation. The only thing I have to go by is that neither the doctor, Henrietta, nor Sharon can feel a lump, and my liver does not feel swollen. Thank you God for these women who have dedicated their lives to helping sick people. I think I am back on track mentally and I can continue fighting.

Dr. George Malkmus sent a health tip on breast cancer for his weekly e-mail called Hallelujah Health Tip. He was quoting the findings of the China Health Project where "researchers found that deaths from breast cancer were associated with five things - high intake of dietary fat, high levels of blood cholesterol, estrogen, and blood testosterone and early age of first menstruation." "In China, we found that relatively small additions to the diet of meat, milk and fat were associated with increasing levels of estrogen and other reproductive hormones." He says, "Hallelujah Acres, for many years has been warning women (and men), that estrogen and animal consumption, were a major cause of breast cancer, as well as numerous other cancers and physical problems! (Many men are also experiencing breast cancer today because of these hormones.)" That confirms to me that being on estrogen blockers and being a vegan is the right thing to do to starve this tumor.

Saturday, August 10, 2002. One thing I've been having a hard time understanding is blood pH. My reports from Sanoviv showed that my blood was very alkaline. Dr. Vazquez explained that this indicated my tissues were very acidic. I believed him but I did not get the physiology behind it. Now, reading the "pH Miracle", I found the clearest explanation: "As mentioned, the ideal blood pH is 7.365. The American medical establishment accepts 7.4, but that is *too* alkaline, and actually indicates tissue acidification. It indicates that the body is collecting and storing alkaline minerals to tame the excess acidity. If it isn't fending off acidity, the body has no need to get so far alkaline." (p 34) The first time I went to Mexico my blood pH was 7.54 and the second time it was 7.46! No wonder cancer was thriving in my body! The foods that are acidic are all the foods I used to eat: meat, dairy and sugar. I would really like to know what my blood pH is now.

Two days ago, my Rife machine arrived from Sanoviv. I have already got it programmed and I'm using the foot plates to receive the frequencies. We just need to get the ray tubes working, so I'll be talking to the biotech guy on Monday. I went on the program for joints and already my pain is decreased!

Monday, August 26, 2002. This last week was extremely emotional. I was feeling so overwhelmed by everything that I started falling apart. Donna was supposed to come for supper last Wed and I was such a basket case I could not even cook anything. I was so convinced I was dying that I got Donna to call dad in Oklahoma. She left a message with his wife that I was having symptoms and would have to go for more tests. Dr. TaI ordered a bone scan for me to make sure there were no bone metastases (cancer spreading to the bone). The tech did tell me there was a lot of degeneration in my joints and Dr. TaI called me Friday night to let me know there was no cancer in the bones.

My garden and yard have been getting full of weeds so Sherree and Donna organized some help to come on Saturday. I struggle so much with asking for help and having energy to organize assistance. How can I ever thank friends like that? I am so grateful.

Dad called me back when he got the message. It is the first time we have spoken in five years. Right now the past does not matter, I just want my dad. He talked to me for about one minute and told me he's hoping for the best for me.

God is Bigger

Saturday, August 31, 2002. Yesterday I was sobbing with relief on the colon hydrotherapy table. I had just found out that my abdominal ultrasound the oncologist ordered was normal. I was concerned about it all week, plus I'm in so much pain from the Zoladex. Sometimes it becomes too much for me. I prayed to God for mercy, to allow me more time here. I thank Him so much for every day that I have. He says in Jeremiah 30:17: "I will give you back your health and heal your wounds." Lord I ask for those words to be a reality in my life. I want to be a blessing to others.

Tuesday, September 3, 2002. Today I saw a biological dentist named Dr. Gary Sacher. He's going to be removing the remaining 5 mercury amalgams in my teeth. His clinic reminded me of Sanoviv and when I met him, I liked him right away. He is familiar with Sanoviv and actually met Dr. Wentz in Germany at a Vega conference. Dr. Sacher described Dr. Wentz as a brilliant man, which of course I agree with. Being the founder of Sanoviv is just one of Dr. Wentz's many accomplishments.

I also saw Henrietta after work and had a follow-up with the Vega Test. I did not tell her that my abdominal ultrasound was clear because I wanted to see what the Vega would read first. It was completely clear, except for my ongoing joint problems, which showed up. Amazing machine. Henrietta told me that she worked with Dr. Sacher for awhile, to help him get set up with the Vega test. Henrietta's own practice became so busy that she could not continue working there, but she spoke very highly of Dr. Sacher.

Sunday, September 8, 2002. I took Allison to see the Imax film, *Jane Goodall's Chimpanzees.* The parkland in Africa looked like paradise.

Sunday, September 15, 2002. Today I woke up with a lot of fear, and I just wanted to be with God. I read in Hebrews 10:35, 36: "So do not throw away your confidence, it will be richly rewarded. You need to persevere so that when you have done the will of God, you will receive what he has promised." After I read that, I made eight cups of carrot/apple/ alfalfa juice. This was a victorious day because I finally succeeded in drinking a full eight cups of juice. On Friday, I got the alfalfa from one of my friends, Doug, who lives on a farm. He gave me a whole bag of apples and when I saw all his alfalfa, I remembered Dr. Norman Walker saying alfalfa was very good for juice, so I asked for a bag of that too. Thank you God and thank you Doug!

Thursday, September 19, 2002. Yesterday, after much begging, I finally got my MRI of the breast. This is a happy day for me because the MRI is normal!!!!! No sign of residual cancer!!! "Praise the Lord who forgives all your sins and heals all your diseases!" (Psalm 103:2,3) Thank you Jesus!!!! I knew You would do it, I just did not know how! I am booked to return to Sanoviv this coming Sunday. I can't wait to give everybody a big hug! It's such a bonus to be able to go back with a good report. So why am I going? Any cancer lumps under one half cm do not show up on an MRI, so I need Dr. Vazquez' advice as to what to do next. So far everything he has told me to do has worked, so if Dr. Vazquez tells me I have to climb a mountain in order to be totally healed, I will. Seriously, I do not know whether I need to continue with Arimidex and Zoladex or if I need something else. It would be great if all I need now is to continue juicing, eating a vegan diet, and all the rest of God's ten-step health plan. No more drugs! The sunlight in Mexico is looking pretty appealing right now, because it is getting darn cold in Edmonton again. Minus 4 Celsius is predicted for Sunday night.

Thursday, October 3, 2002. I gave myself a homeopathic injection, had a severe allergic reaction and had to go to emergency. I was given reactin, epinephrine and a steroid to get rid of the rash, the constriction in my throat and the swelling.

Friday, October 4, 2002. Now that unpleasant episode is over I can write about more uplifting things. I was very encouraged during my visit to Sanoviv last week. On the plane down there I was so excited about my MRI results that I was telling the two business men next to me all about Sanoviv. They were pretty interested. Then I was met at the San Diego airport by the smiling van driver, Mauricio, who takes guests across the border. In the van were two girls from Michigan and a couple from New Mexico who were gourmet live food chefs. One of the girls, Monica, was also a breast cancer patient and we shared our stories. After she heard my story she was really glad she was on her way to Sanoviv.

Upon arrival at the retreat, the intake doctor took a complete history and did a thorough examination. Then it was supper time (sprout time). After supper, forms have to be filled out for all the departments because they have a meeting first thing in the morning. Dental, Psychological, Spa, Fitness, Medical - hard to fill them all out when you are wiped from travelling, but worth it. Saliva and urine have to be taken down to the lab at 7 a.m. and blood work done. The Bioenergetics department did all kinds of testing in the morning, then darkfield microscopic work was done. A dental evaluation, fitness evaluation and psychological consult consumed the afternoon. After that they scheduled a relaxing pedicure. In the one hour of free time I enjoyed the thalasso (salt water) pool.

I was happy with my fitness evaluation - I've gone from poor to fair as far as percentage of body fat. It is now down to 29 per cent. In a few months I'll be good, which would be 24-27%. One year ago I was 39% so that is great progress. I tested with excellent breathing capacity, average strength, above average cardiovascular fitness level and normal flexibility. Still work to do with stretching - I have to get a Swiss ball.

A decision was made that I would stay on the Zoladex for 3 more months, then another MRI should be done to make sure we are still on the right track. Dr. Vazquez gave me some meds that took care of the joint pain so I agreed to stay on Zoladex. I still will continue with colon therapy, massage and MRT (Matrix Regeneration Therapy). MRT is now available at Henrietta's clinic.

Wednesday, October 9, 2002. This has been a rewarding week. Saturday I spent two hours with Denise, showing her some of the things I have learned over the past year, like how to sprout and how to juice. Denise and I went to church in the evening. I thanked her pastor for praying for me last year, then he asked me to come and testify on Sunday morning. When I was coming back from Mexico, I had a strong impression that I was supposed to be sharing with as many churches as possible how God has led me through this trial. When I shared on Sunday, I emphasized the book *Christ the Healer* and the *Back to the Garden diet.*

Yesterday I made a "living food" salad for Allison and myself. It was an Arame salad with mung bean sprouts. Arame is a type of sea vegetable that comes in strips about the thickness of spaghetti. It is mild tasting and is a good way to introduce someone to sea vegetables. It only has to be soaked for about 15 minutes before it is ready to use.

Monday, October 14, 2002. Today I did another consultation for two hours. So many people are asking me for information about how to prevent disease, I decided to start charging for it. This way I can slowly pay off my loan for medical expenses. Part of the price includes the organic juice and the wear and tear on the videos and books. Denise told me today, she wants to keep the videos and book I lent her for longer because they are so incredible. There is so much information in them that you cannot absorb it all in one week.

Revenue Canada sent me a letter saying that they will not accept my receipts for colon hydrotherapy, massage therapy or the alternative health clinic because they "are not recognized as medical practitioners in the province where [I] received the services". Revenue Canada wants me to pay back part of my income tax return. I was so devastated by that letter that I couldn't deal with it for days. I spent $29,000 on medical expenses last year and only less than $8,000 was returned to me. Now they want part of that back. This is a country that is supposed to cover our medical expenses. Part of the treatments at Sanoviv were not covered, i.e., the massage therapy. I did not even send in my receipts from the pharmacy in Sanoviv because I assumed the entire stay was way over the amount allowed for deduction. Since substances "prescribed by a medical practitioner and dispensed and recorded by a pharmacist" are deductible, I will now send them. It is just sad to me that preventive treatments are not covered, only pharmaceutical treatments.

Complementary medicine has come a long way over the years, as far as being recognized, but I can see there is still a long way to go. It is well known by the medical establishment that most people are loaded with fecal matter and that constipation can lead to the formation of pockets (diverticuli), but they will not recognise colon hydrotherapy! Is it because there is too much money to be made selling laxatives, doing colon surgery, and running tests on colons? If the pharmaceutical industry does in fact control what doctors learn in medical school, which would explain why none of them know about colon hydrotherapy.

Wednesday, October 16, 2002. I just found out from the Alternative Health Clinic that many people have submitted their receipts with their income tax returns and they have been accepted. They write a letter that includes the paragraph: "Because I practice preventive health care for myself I am remitting the enclosed receipts as medical expenses. I am of the opinion that my choice to be responsible for my own health has saved health care costs and has reduced the burden on the health care system." So I am giving it a try.

Saturday, October 19, 2002. Donna, Ivan and I went for a long walk in the river valley. It was a calm, misty day, perfect for walking. I am really praying about where God wants to take me with what I've learned. I know He is big.

Thursday, October 24, 2002. I saw my oncologist on Tuesday. He told me he knows my cancer is going to come back. He stated there is no evidence that what I am doing works. (I think that's because there have been no large 'official' studies done) He also said I am lasting longer than he thought I would. Without denying the seriousness of the situation I am in, that really makes me laugh! He really contributed to my humor therapy this week.

I ordered *The Miraculous Self-Healing Body* video from Hallelujah Acres as I seem to have an ongoing need for inspiration.

Friday, November 1, 2002. So many things are happening. The fellow I did a consultation with a few weeks ago is so excited about what he has learned that he started referring people to me. He can't wait to get more material. That is really rewarding to me. I pray that this wave will continue and grow until there are people all over catching the vision.

I had a live blood analysis done today. The red cells were showing a bit of stress, but I also had good healing potential, so in other words the blood cells are dealing with the stress that they have. They did not show the characteristics of cancer, which is a good sign. The white blood cells looked healthy and appeared to be doing a good clean up job. I had to get some evening primrose oil in order to improve the strength and the shape of the red blood cells. The nurse who did the analysis commended me on my hard work, because one year ago my blood analysis at Sanoviv was a mess. I would really recommend people have this done, because it tells you a lot about what is going on in your body.

Another new thing that has happened is that I went to a Seventh Day Adventist church last Sunday evening. The church is having a series of teachings for a few weeks, almost every night of the week, so I will be going again tonight. It was really encouraging to talk to the pastor, because he is so passionate about the vegan/ Garden of Eden lifestyle. Other people at the church were the same way. The funny thing is that I have worked right next door to that church for 15 years and now I'm finally entering it! As I mentioned earlier, I had always been taught negative things about Seventh Day Adventism. I am happy to learn they are doing so many good things in the area of health. For example, one Adventist couple have a ministry in Lavoy Alberta where people go to get detoxed. That sounds like something for drug addicts, but it is actually more for junk food addicts!

Saturday, November 2, 2002. Yesterday I made some Essiac tea. This tea was developed by a Canadian nurse named Rene Caisse in the 1920s and is actually her last name spelled backwards. Essiac tea has burdock (anti-tumor properties), slippery elm herb (a cleanser), sheep sorrel (inhibits chromosome damage), and rhubarb root (expels wastes). It is a very good adjunctive therapy no matter what cancer treatment one may be taking. The tea is prepared over a period of a day and is ready to drink the next day. Because you only drink a couple of ounces every 12 hours, the tea lasts quite awhile. Now that my tumor is gone, I want to keep it that way. With God's help, I will never go back to old habits.

Denise called today and she's very excited about her new Champion juicer. She was also interested in a dry skin brush, which helps to stimulate the lymphatic system. I got a couple of brushes down in Sanoviv and sold her one. Lightly brushing on the surface of the skin, always towards the heart, helps to move the lymphatic fluid along. When they talked about it in detox class, I thought it was pretty strange to brush your skin, but now I try to do it as much as I can. It is so neat what God is doing - we're all learning about the bodies that He gave us, and they are truly miraculous.

At my weekly trip to the farmer's market to buy carrots today, I ran into my friend Jim and we ended up going for a walk for about an hour. It was a beautiful sunny day. It felt nice to have a friend to walk with.

Sunday, November 3, 2002. This morning was a fun day at children's church. We divided the children into groups and had different stations for them to visit. The theme was Afghanistan because this year Samaritan's Purse is sending shoe boxes to various countries and Afghanistan is one of them. I brought some bread typical of Afghanistan and showed them the DarI alphabet. Everybody took home a shoe box to fill for a needy child.

This evening I made dinner for Stewart and his wife Penny. Stewart has been faithfully coming and juicing for me for months now and I am very grateful. I tried a new way to cook brussel sprouts that I learned from Dr. Day's video. You put diced onion in the bottom of a pot, turn the heat on minimum, put the vegetables on top of the onions and let them heat up slowly for about an hour. This way the cell membranes of the vegetable do not burst and you do not lose nutrients to the water, because there is no water. Cooking this way works well for things like cauliflower and broccoli, but not as well for hard vegetables like beets. Of course, the best way to eat vegetables is raw, but I do not eat everything raw right now, especially in winter.

Tuesday, November 5, 2002. I just gave myself a mistletoe injection. In September, Dr. Vazquez gave me a two-month supply so I inject half a vial into the breast and half into my arm.

If there is any cancer cells left in there, I don't know how they would have a chance with all the things they are being hit with.

Lan, the fellow who came to my house for a consultation, now has a vision to turn his home into a healing centre. As a chiropractor, he is already sharing Dr. Day's videos with his patients. He told me that he believes God allowed me to go through this trial so that I could help other people. Even though I could not see what He was doing when I was diagnosed, I knew He was up to something. God is bigger!

Getting More Disciplined

Saturday, November 9, 2002. I have been listening to Dr. George Malkmus' audiotape *How to Eliminate Sickness*. What an inspired man he is. His comments on estrogen really struck me because I have found the statements to be so true in my own life. He said that breast cancer is largely a disease caused by estrogen and that if we could eliminate estrogen from women's bodies we would virtually eliminate breast cancer. That is a very radical statement but it is exactly what happened to me. When the doctors at Sanoviv put me on Zoladex, this stopped the production of estrogen in my body. I chose to do that because of the aggressiveness of my cancer. However, if I had been a vegan all my life, I would have had less body fat and hence less estrogen. My breasts would not have gotten as large as they did over the last decade. I just want to tell all the women in the world: if you're putting on weight, get off animal products! Even if you're not putting on weight, get off them! Dr. Malkmus has a lengthy teaching on estrogen in one of his weekly *Hallelujah health tips* which are sent via email.

Sunday, November 10, 2002. After church, Cyril and Cathy came over bringing bags of raw vegetables and fruit. We sat and munched on veggies. The veggies were totally satisfying even without any dip. Cyril and Cathy have been vegetarian for quite awhile now and both have lost a lot of weight, especially cutting out cheese. Cyril's cholesterol has dropped several points. I thank God for friends like Cyril and Cathy whom I have known for a long time.

Monday, November 11, 2002. Today I wrote an article for a local newspaper on my experience with breast cancer. I pray it will be accepted so that women will know that they have options.

Wednesday, November 13, 2002. The director of the Cancer Institute made a decision *not* to cover my Zoladex. The Cross Institute will give me Zoladex but I have to pay for it myself to the tune of $500 per month. The reason? I have not had a treatment failure with tamoxifen. Instead, I am taking arimidex which studies show gives far better results than tamoxifen. Why are they still giving tamoxifen to women? It boils down to money. It costs only about 50 cents per pill, whereas arimidex is over

$4 per pill. How many more women have to experience "treatment failures" with tamoxifen before the cancer institute will change their policy?

Sunday, November 17, 2002. Teresa and I had a big plate of raw vegetables for lunch. Very satisfying. It's good to receive the nutrients from the earth through our food. I was just introduced to Dr. Bernard Jensen's work this weekend and he says: "We are made from the dust of the earth... We do not eat earth per se. But, we do consume it in a transmuted form through vegetables, fruits and so forth."[27] Dr. Jensen was a chiropractor who turned to the art of nutrition in search of remedies for his own health problems. He travelled to over 50 countries to study the lifestyles of long-lived peoples. This led him to places like Russia and to Pakistan where the Hunza's live.

I have been thinking for awhile that I need to get more disciplined with my food. To most people it already seems like I am extremely disciplined but I just spoke with a lady that I took a living foods course from, and she pinpointed some areas that I need to improve on. Connie told me it is good that I'm not eating meat or dairy or sugar but I need to get rid of my becel margarine and only use flax oil, Udo's oil or avocado. Also I have been eating nan bread for a couple of weeks now and that is an absolute no-no. Eating white flour is just like eating sugar. She told me that until she got really strict with her diet that her fibroid tumor would not go away. I know these things from being at Sanoviv but that is one area that I've been compromising on. With this disease you cannot slip up in one area or the tumor won't budge. Connie shared with me that with or without medication she would do everything possible diet-wise to beat the cancer. Becel and nan bread are going out the door!

Sunday, November 24, 2002. Ellen G. White's writings are blowing me away. One of the pastors at the Seventh Day Adventist church gave me her *Counsels on Diet and Foods* and I am amazed at the wisdom that God gave her, as well as the volume of writing that she did. This was written in 1905: "If men today were simple in their habits, living in harmony with nature's laws, as did Adam and Eve in the beginning, there would be an abundant supply for the needs of the human family. But selfishness and the indulgence of appetite have brought sin and misery, from excess on the one hand, and from want on the other." (p 91)[28] How true!

The Seventh Day Adventists have pot lucks after their service on Saturday. These pot lucks are totally vegetarian. Yesterday I was there because a friend was getting baptised and also because I am thinking of changing churches. I notice that the people vary in their degrees of vegetarianism. Some of them eat cheese and eggs and some even do eat a small amount of meat (but not at the Sabbath meal). They do put sugar in some of their dishes, which I think is because not all of them have completely received the health message. Anyway, I can sure handle their potlucks better than the ones at my present church. There is not only an ignorance of the importance of proper diet, there seems to be an active resistance to learning anything. The first thing you see and smell when you walk into the church I attend on Sunday, is coffee, the Christian drug.

Tuesday, November 26, 2002. Listening to George Malkmus' audiotape "How to Eliminate Sickness" has motivated me to start having Barley Green for breakfast. Dr. Malkmus has had Barley Green for breakfast for over 25 years and he says he is full of energy all morning long. You just mix a tablespoon of the powder in a couple of ounces of water. It really does not taste bad, in fact it is much better than wheatgrass. I have his tape in the car and I listen to it over and over when I'm driving anywhere.

Thursday, November 27, 2002. I woke up at 5 a.m. ready to go, just like Rev Malkmus. (Actually I think he's up at 4 a.m. but 5 is really good for me!) Had lemon water and rebounded for 10 minutes. I have a colon therapy session today and the therapist wants me to drink peppermint tea to cut down on intestinal gas, so I am doing that. Hopefully we will get further up the colon in our session today.

Counsels on Diet and Foods continues to inspire me. In the chapter on over-eating E. White writes: "... surplus food burdens the system, and produces morbid, feverish conditions. It calls an undue amount of blood to the stomach, causing limbs and extremities to chill quickly." (p 134) A totally novel idea as to why so many patients of ours complain of cold hands and feet, something that used to bother me a lot. The statement I really like is: "While sitting at the table we may do medical missionary work by eating and drinking to the glory of God." That really touches me because all of my Christian life, I have been involved in medical missionary work but because of my illness I have been unable to travel overseas these past couple of years. Now I can be involved in medical missions right where I am. Wow!

Tuesday, December 3, 2002. I watched two videotapes of testimonials from Hallelujah Acres. A couple of doctors testified how the Hallelujah diet had healed their health problems; one of them had a lung tumor the size of a grapefruit. Another one, Dr. Chesnut, expressed remorse that he had missed so many years that he could have spent helping people if he had known about the connection between diet and disease. He said that because he was told in medical school that diet did not matter, he told his patients that diet did not matter. Now as a retired doctor, Dr. Chesnut voluntarily helps people, because he's "sick and tired of doctors profiting off of vulnerable people."[29]

Friday, December 6, 2002. As part of my devotional I am still reading Ellen White's Councils on Diet and Foods. This is what she wrote in 1900: "There are many now under the shadow of death who have prepared to do a work for the Master but who have not felt a sacred obligation rested upon them to observe the laws of health. The laws of the physical system are indeed the laws of God; but this fact seems to have been forgotten." (p 212) She amazes me.

Saturday, December 7, 2002. This is what Ellen White wrote in 1875: "Many mothers who deplore the intemperance which exists everywhere, do not look deep enough to see the cause. They are daily preparing a variety of dishes and highly seasoned food, which tempt the appetite and encourage overeating. ...Flesh meats constitute the principal article of food upon the tables of some families, until their blood is filled with cancerous and scrofulous humors."(p 233) She really has wisdom.

It is the Sabbath today. I have been going to church on Saturday for about a month now. I feel so much more peaceful since I've been doing that, and I have met quite a few friendly people there. I did not realize that the day of worship for Christians was always Saturday until the Catholic church changed it to Sunday. Since my way of living lines up with the 7th Day Adventists, maybe I should change my day for corporate worship too!

Sunday, December 8, 2002. I had lunch with Teresa today then we went for a walk. Tonight I am continuing to soak up Ellen White's teaching. In 1902, she made this remarkable statement: "Animals are becoming more and more diseased, and it will not be long until animal food will be discarded by many besides Seventh-day Adventists. Foods that are healthful and life sustaining are to be prepared, so that men and women will not need to eat meat." (p 267) That is exactly what is happening! Places like Sanoviv and Hallelujah Acres are springing up around the world.

Monday, December 16, 2002. Donna and I went for a 2-hour walk on Saturday then we put together a meal of salad, lentils, rice and corn bread. That was fun cooking together. On Sunday evening we went out to a little country church near New Sarepta Alberta to hear a guest speaker. The pastor spoke with me afterward and he really encouraged me. I told him what I have been dealing with for the past two years and how I have changed my lifestyle. He asked me if I had ever heard of the Hallelujah Acres diet! I was so thrilled that he had heard of it and has incorporated many of the principles into his life. Pastor Marvin told me that he spent a couple of months teaching the Hallelujah diet and he lost half his congregation over it! However, he really felt that God wanted him to teach the Hallelujah lifestyle and does not feel it was in vain. What really encouraged me was that he feels God is going to use what I am going through to help many people. I know that depends on me - whether or not I remain disciplined and whether or not I keep close to God.

The reason I am saying that is it is the Christmas season and there is an awful lot of chocolate around. People keep bringing chocolates to the office and I have been into it for 3 days now. I'm ok on the weekends because I can control the environment but I cannot control my work environment. What I am saying is: God I'm weak, help me in my weakness. I want to be like Paul the apostle: "Therefore I do not run like a man running aimlessly; I do not fight like a man beating the air. No, I beat my body and make it my slave so that after I have preached to others, I myself will not be disqualified for the prize." (1Cor 9: 26, 27) Of course he does not really beat his body; he is talking about discipline!

Wednesday, December 18, 2002. Since I had that talk with God on Monday, I have been doing much better. No chocolate for two days. God, keep helping me!

Dr. Bernard Jensen motivated me to do my dry skin brushing today. I read in his book, *A New Lifestyle for Health and Happiness:* "The skin eliminates two pounds of toxic waste each day. These uric acid crystals, catarrh and various other acids are more easily eliminated when the top layer of dead skin is removed. The skin [is] a "third" kidney because it helps get rid of uric acid to relieve the work of the kidneys which normally get rid of two lbs of waste daily." (p 29) When you understand what is going on you have a lot more incentive to do something that otherwise seems a bit silly. I have been brushing my skin sometimes but I did not quite have the whole picture.

Sunday, December 29, 2002. I awoke up at 6:00 a.m. today. That happens to me all the time now that I am not taking antidepressants. I have already had my lemon water, done the dishes, done some vacuuming, got supper started, watched a one hour video, and had breakfast and it's only 9 a.m. I love having all this energy in the morning.

I had some awesome blessings this Christmas. Kim told me I could keep the champion juicer that she's been lending me all year. That just blew me away because it's worth $400. Allison got me a gift certificate for the organic market, my sister Jennifer got me some organic food and mom got me a gift certificate to go buy some new size 12 clothes! I'm still getting rid of size 16's. My dad was here for a few days and he did not want to see me and that made me sad, but God provided a safe place for me to go on Christmas evening when he arrived at my sister's. It was a really neat family named the Flickingers who live out on an acreage. The Flickingers open their home on Christmas day for people. I was able to talk to them about what God has been doing in my life and it encouraged me because they knew about the Hallelujah Acres diet and even had George Malkmus' book.

On Boxing Day some singles from the Christian Friendship Circle came over and we walked and sang and had a meal together. I felt so blessed to have such beautiful friends.

Monday, December 30, 2002. My friend Donna came over yesterday and we went for a walk. She helped me make eight cups of carrot juice. What an awesome friend. She is so interested in learning about this wonderful lifestyle that God has led me to.

"Cancers, tumors and all inflammatory diseases are largely caused by meat eating." I just read that in Ellen White's book. She wrote it in 1896! "Those who use flesh meats freely, do not always have an unclouded brain and an active intellect, because the use of the flesh of animals tends to cause a grossness of body, and to benumb the finer sensibilities of the mind." (1890) What is so amazing about her statements is that they are being confirmed now by people like Dr. Klaper, Dr. John McDougal, Dr. George Malkmus, and Dr. Lorraine Day. This is what she wrote in 1875: "Flesh meats constitute the principle article of food upon the tables of some families, until their blood is filled with cancerous and scrofulous humors. Their bodies are composed of what they eat. But when suffering and disease come upon them, it is considered an affliction of Providence." It seems as if very little has changed in 125 years!

Wednesday, January 1, 2003. Wow, I brought in the New Year in an awesome way! Pastor Marvin Swanson invited me to the New Sarepta Country Church to share my testimony. People were so receptive. Several of them are already planning to do a "Daniel fast," which is the diet that Daniel in the Old Testament requested while he was in Babylon. Instead of the rich food that he was being offered, he asked for vegetables and water, and he ended up healthier than the royalty. Because Pastor Marvin stated publicly that he believes in the Hallelujah Acres diet, I think that a very strong relationship is going to be built between his family and myself.

The rest of the New Year's Eve service consisted of worship and people giving testimonies. I did not get home till 3:00 this morning so today was a recuperation day. It was a beautiful sunny day for walking.

Thursday, January 2, 2003. "By precept and example make it plain that the food, which God gave Adam in his sinless state is the best for man's use as he seeks to regain that sinless state." (p460, Ellen White) A good reminder to eat raw food. Tomorrow I am going to eat mostly raw. Today, I ate mostly cooked and I can feel the effect. Cooked food is more acidic than raw food and we know we do not want our tissues to be in an acidic state.

Saturday, January 4, 2003. "The science of cooking is not a small matter. The skillful preparation of food is one of the most essential arts. It should be regarded as among the most valuable of all the arts, because it is so closely connected with the life." (p 475, Ellen White) That truth is becoming more and more a part of my life.

Donna came over today and we prepared a lunch together. We made a meatless loaf and a rainbow salad full of red cabbage, beets, squash, peppers, lettuce, cucumbers and sprouts. She is the fourth person I've done a consultation with and it is such a joy because she appreciates everything so much. That meatless loaf is a real blessing because it satisfies the same way as meatloaf would without all the damage that meat does.

Sunday, January 5, 2003. "Remember this: God is the ruler, God is the healer, but nature is the garment around God. We can touch His garment in the green vegetables - the fresh asparagus, the ripe apricots, the bloom on the cheek of the peach."[30] Thank you God for carrot-spinach juice! One of my favorite Bible verses is: "They begged him to let them touch even the hem of his garment and *all* who touched him were healed." (Mark 6:56) I never thought of his garment being the vegetables - what beautiful poetry! If his garment is vegetation, then *all* who want to be healed need to be eating vegetables everyday.

Tuesday, January 7, 2003. The last two mornings I have been up at 5 a.m. making carrot juice. I make 6 cups and take it to work to drink in between meals. Then Stewart comes in the afternoon and makes a couple more cups.

Friday, January 24, 2003. Boy did I crash. I guess I am not George Malkmus. I got really tired and run down and ended up with a bad cold, which has forced me to rest all week. I am just starting to feel better.

Reading Dr. Bernard Jensen today, I learned that celery juice is really good for the joints so I am putting celery in the carrot juice now. "Celery juice is high in organic sodium which helps keep calcium in solution." (p40)[31] "When you go to the doctor and he says the joints are getting stiff because you are getting old, that's not entirely correct. Your joints are getting stiff because sodium is lacking in the joints. (p61) I double-checked the information with Dr. Norman Walker and he also recommended celery juice for arthritis.

Saturday, February 1, 2003. We are experiencing some nice weather for this time of year, so I have been enjoying some good walks this week. Unfortunately, the only part of our body that gets exposed to the sunlight in our Canadian winters is the face.

I'm still into reading Bernard Jensen. He calls wheat one of the six nutritional sins of civilization. "Twenty-nine percent of the American diet - almost one third of our food intake each day - is wheat. This is an outrageous percentage of wheat consumption! Wheat should comprise only 6 per cent of our diet. Wheat contains gluten, which causes a breakdown of the villI in the small intestine. Gluten is responsible for the elasticity in bread dough. Gluten also adheres to the bowel in the same sticky manner." (p96) Keeping wheat consumption down to 6 per cent is another challenge to face in our society. Fortunately, there is an organic store near my house where I can get spelt bread or rye bread. Spelt is a grain that has less gluten then wheat.

Last weekend, I was blessed to be able to go to Jasper with a friend. We had massages, soaked in the hot pool, sat in the steam room and went for a swim in the outdoor pool. Sunday a chinook came through and we had a balmy +6° Celcius. We went for a walk around Pyramid Lake island before heading home. I was feeling pretty upbeat after that wonderful break.

Monday, February 3, 2003. Sometimes it feels like I am at war with cancer 24 hours a day. If I let my guard down for just a little while it pounces like someone quietly waiting in ambush. The last couple of days my breast has started to feel a bit harder again and it has had the orange peel texture, just the way inflammatory breast cancer manifests. I thought: what have I been slacking off on? So I got some more oncolyn because I had stopped taking it, doubled up on my Wobe Mugos, did a coffee enema, and had an MRT (Matrix Regeneration Therapy). I also started hitting the enemy with scripture verses. It really is a war, and every day I need to ask God for the desire to keep fighting. Today I feel like fighting but some days I want somebody else to fight for me. Stewart *still* comes and makes carrot juice but nobody comes on Saturdays and I did not feel like doing it so I did not get any. It doesn't matter what I *feel* like, the enemy is there and if I want to live, I have to fight.

Thursday, February 6, 2003. All week I have been doing coffee enemas. They really seem to help. After doing a regular enema, a weak solution of coffee is implanted into the rectum and descending colon. The coffee travels via the portal vein to the liver and this stimulates the liver to dump toxins. It is controversial. Dr. Day does not recommend it because she found the caffeine was getting into the rest of the body. I have not made up my mind about whether coffee enemas are good or bad. Sanoviv recommended that I do them to detoxify my liver.

This Sunday, I am looking forward to going to Lavoy. I am going to the Abundant Life Therapy Centre for a 10 day cleanse and education retreat.

Abundant Life Therapy Centre

I heard about the Abundant Life Therapy Centre from Irma, a friend in the Seventh Day Adventist church. The results the Abundant Life Therapy Centre is getting with cancer, diabetes, arthritis, weight loss, heart disease and other diseases are nothing short of phenomenal. This is accomplished at very low cost, which makes it affordable to those who cannot go to a place like Sanoviv. Having exhausted my line of credit, I am now among those who cannot afford to go to Sanoviv right now. The Abundant Life Therapy Centre is run by Rudy and Jeannie Davis.

Sunday, February 9, 2003. We had Homozon before going to bed. Homozon is magnesium and oxygen. It is followed by lemon juice which separates the oxygen from the magnesium. This is to prepare us for the isotonic drink in the morning.

Monday, February 10, 2003. 7:30 a.m. All seven of us guests drank two litres of isotonic drink made with celtic sea salt and water. We had to down it all within 20 minutes so it would go completely through the digestive tract without being absorbed. The body instinctively wants to get salt water out as fast as possible but the concentration is too low to induce vomiting so it goes straight through, cleansing built up toxic waste as it goes. Every morning for eight days we drink this.

8:30 a.m. 2 litres of water to be finished by 11 a.m.

9:00 a.m. Liver-gall bladder cleanse. A glass of fresh orange juice mixed with a tablespoon of olive oil and a clove of garlic. Every day for an additional four days the garlic is increased.

9:30 a.m. Shot of Wheatgrass with apples. Most of us experience a hard time with wheatgrass juice but the apples help. Wheatgrass juice is one of the best sources of living chlorophyll available. Dr. Bernard Jensen says it only takes minutes to digest wheat grass juice. The juice also helps purify the liver among many other things. I started reading the "Sproutman's" book on wheatgrass. Steve Meyerowitz is known as the sproutman because of his innovative ideas on preparing food with sprouts.

10:00 a.m. Worship and devotions led by Rudy Davis. The health message comes through loud and clear in the bible. Psalm 119:71

- "It was good for me to be afflicted so that I might learn your decrees." vs 67 - "Before I was afflicted I went astray but now I obey your word." vs 92 - "If your law had not been my delight, I would have perished in my affliction." We need to follow the diet God gave us in the Garden of Eden or we will end up with all kinds of afflictions. Our living body needs living food. Many times I have thought that God was allowing me to be afflicted so that I might grow closer to Him and learn the lifestyle He planned for us humans.

12:30 p.m. Poultice drink made of fresh apple juice, charcoal, psyllium, marshmallow root and other cleansing ingredients. We get this twice a day for 5 days to help loosen built up fecal matter.

1:00 p.m. Walk for at least 45 minutes around the big town of Lavoy (pop 65).

2:00 p.m. 2 litres of water to be finished by 6 pm.

2:30 p.m. Shot of wheatgrass with apples. Lots of funny faces.

3:15 p.m. Walk for 30 minutes.

3:45 p.m. Health lecture. *Why will you die O house of Israel?* Believers belong to Israel in the spiritual sense and many of them are perishing for lack of knowledge. God's ideal diet is vegan but very few Christians know this.

Plants do something that no animal can do - take the minerals out of the soil and make them usable to us. The plant is able to attach a protein enzyme to the minerals in the earth and make them organic.

It is impossible for the liver to digest uric acid, which comes from animals. Uric acid causes Parkinsons. People with Parkinsons who go on a raw food diet stop the shaking. Rudy told us that the human body is smarter than we know and smarter than we can know.

5:00 p.m. Worship.

5:55 p.m. Poultice drink. (Draws toxins off the inside of digestive tract)

6:00 p.m. Steam bath. 15 minutes in the steam room followed by 30 seconds in the cold shower. Do this 3 times. This will increase your lymphocyte count to 40,000. If you lay down for half an hour afterwards, it will temporarily increase to 60,000. You can do major damage to cancer cells and other unwanted invaders!

8:00 p.m. Lights out.

I just want to say to anyone reading this that the program needs to be administered by a trained person because some people may have special considerations. For example there was one lady in our program who did not partake in all the drinks because of risk to her fragile system. She was on a modified program. Rudy and Jeannie have both taken extensive training in California and are both working on their doctorates in naturopathy under Dr. Joel Robbins. These drinks should not be taken here and there, but are designed to work together over the 10-day period.

Tuesday, February 11, 2003. I learned some interesting things in the health lecture on colon care by Jeannie. One thing that struck me was that the human body runs on carbohydrates. This is converted to sugar. It is very hard for the body to turn protein to sugar. In fact, it will use fat before it will use protein. All the protein diets that you hear about are extremely dangerous.

Another eye-opening fact is that we produce four to six cups of saliva and two and one half gallons of gastric juice per day. We use 40,000 cups of water per day but only lose eight cups because the rest are recycled during all the functions the body performs.

This is why it is so important not to lie down after you eat: you can get a hiatal hernia! The pressure caused by lying down with a full stomach pushes the stomach upwards! The simple cure for this is to drink a gallon of water and jump off a step three times. I am sure that any surgery-happy doctor reading this is laughing his/her head off by now but if you have a hiatal hernia try it! (And stop eating before you go to bed!)

Here is another reason not to use dairy products: they plug up the opening from the appendix, leading to appendicitis.

We learned a horrifying fact in our video lecture by Dr. Joel Robbins: The average American goes 14 days without eating any fresh fruits or vegetables! Since fruits and vegetables are the only foods that can keep our body tissues alkaline, the average American is extremely acidic, the perfect environment for cancer to thrive in. Cancer cannot exist in a cell pH of 5.7 or higher. The blood pH always needs to be 7.4. If it goes down to 7.2 we will die, so if the pH level starts to drop, the blood will take alkaline minerals from the body in order to maintain the right balance. If you cook raw fruits and vegetables, they become less alkaline than they are in the uncooked state so that is why it is so crucial to eat them raw.

Another amazing fact from Dr. Joel Robbins is that in cities where doctors' strikes occurred, the death rate dropped! I guess if doctors are not around to prescribe drugs to suppress symptoms, people have to deal with the root cause of their problem. (Of course there are times when the only thing that will save a person's life is a drug.) Dr. Robbins teaches that the symptom is our friend; it is our body telling us that we need to take care of something. Cancer is the body's last-ditch attempt to tell us we have to make changes; it is the end disease of all diseases. As horrible as cancer is, it is actually our body's way of prolonging our life. If we take care of the cause, the cancer will go away, that is if we get to it before it has consumed our entire body.

If we put too many toxins into our body, our liver becomes congested. It will eventually kick the toxins out into the blood stream, then the cells will have to release alkaline material to neutralize the toxins. The liver can only deal with the toxins when the body becomes more alkaline.

Those were the things I learned from Dr. Joel Robbins, who apparently worked quite extensively with Dr. Lorraine Day when she first got sick.

Thursday, February 13, 2003. Rudy gave a lecture on water retention. He taught us that when our tissues are full of toxins water moves in to the tissues to separate the toxins so they do not enter the cells. Lymphatic clogging is because the lymph system is trying to do its work. A lymph node has only one exit, but many channels where matter can enter. Since it can only handle one toxin at a time, it becomes clogged when there are many unwanted substances in the system. It is a main factor in inflammatory breast cancer.

We also learned the three 8-hour cycles that our body should run on. From 12 p.m. - 8 p.m. we are digesting, from 8 p.m. - 4 a.m. we are assimilating, and from 4 a.m. - 12 p.m. we are eliminating. So the three cycles are Digestion, Assimilation and Elimination. This is why the optimal time to be in bed is 8 p.m. I have noticed that in most places in the world 8 p.m. is when people go to bed because they don't have any artificial light to see by. Nature is a lot smarter than we are with all our brilliant technology!

Friday, February 14, 2003. We listened to George Malkmus on video speaking at the 4th Prophesy Conference. He urged us to "present your bodies a living sacrifice and be not conformed to this world." (Rom12:1,2) Not being conformed to the world includes the way that we eat. The average American puts 12 pounds of chemical preservatives into the diet every year but the person who does this will only be presenting a half dead sacrifice to the Lord!

For the afternoon lecture we heard Dr. Hans Diehl sharing about his 30 day C.H.I.P. program, or the Coronary Health Improvement Project. I am actually registered to start that program on February 23, 2003. My cholesterol usually runs around 6 - 6.5. Dr. Diehl told us that a reading of 6.5 compared to 5.5 raises the risk of heart disease 400%! Lowering the cholesterol levels could not hurt in the fight against cancer as well. We accept 5.2 as normal in Canada (around 200 in the States) but Dr. Diehl said the best cholesterol is 100 + your age (lower than 4 in Canada). Vegans have no dietary source of cholesterol, which is good, but they can still get high cholesterol from putting too much fat in the diet. The vegetable fat stimulates the liver to produce cholesterol. There are no recorded cases of heart attacks in people with cholesterol levels under 150 mg per cent!

Tuesday, February 18, 2003. Dane and VickI Griffin spoke on *The Great Sugar Scandal*, through video. Only six teaspoons of sugar will decrease your body's immune system by 25 per cent, 12 teaspoons decrease it by 60 per cent, 18 teaspoons bring it down by 85 per cent and 25 teaspoons decrease it by 92 per cent. The average American consumes 35 teaspoons per day so they are virtually shutting down their immune systems. VickI suggested putting sugar in the toilet bowl. It makes a good cleaner!

Saturday, March 1, 2003. I came away from The Abundant Life Therapy Centre with greatly increased faith. I have new ideas about how to prepare the beautiful fruits, seeds and vegetables that God has provided for us. One thing I have always loved is halvah and I learned how to make it! It is so simple to make out of ground sesame seeds and a natural sweetener like brown rice syrup.

After reading *The Wheatgrass Book* by Steve Myerowitz I am much more faithful about taking Barley Max. He talks in detail about the benefits of not only wheatgrass but also barley grass.[33] I cannot seem to fit fresh wheat grass into my schedule so I do the next best thing and shake up powdered Barley Max in a jar. Barley Max is Hallelujah Acres new green drink made from barley greens and alfalfa. It is much easier to get down than wheatgrass, as it does not induce nausea. (Wheatgrass has that effect on me and several other people I have met.) At Abundant Life Therapy Centre we had apples with the wheatgrass, which seemed to cut the nausea for most of us.

Increase the Raw Food!

Saturday, March 15, 2003. Since I started the C.H.I.P. program (the Coronary Health Improvement Project), almost no writing has taken place. We meet from Monday to Thursday evening for two and one half hours each time. It is great teaching and they do wonderful food demonstrations, but I hardly have time to relax! I enrolled in the program because my cholesterol is still high even though I have been vegan for over a year. I found out that consuming too much oil, even if it is vegetable oil, could stimulate the liver to produce cholesterol. This may be a reason for my problem, so I have cut down on the oil. We will see at the end of the course when they retake our blood.

Sunday, March 16, 2003. The C.H.I.P. volunteers have demonstrated many dishes such as vegan enchiladas and vegan lasagna. One of the things I have learned is how to make 8-grain cereal in the crockpot so it's ready to eat first thing in the morning. Most of the food the volunteers do is cooked so it is not quite as "evolved" as the Abundant Life Therapy Centre or Sanoviv as far as reversing a serious illness like cancer but it's great to have these recipes for when you do want something cooked. Eating mostly raw vegan food is still the fastest way to heal from a serious illness and the best way to maintain optimal health.

Sherree and Jim and I went for a walk this afternoon. Now that it has warmed up to zero Celsius a person actually feels like going outside. (Last week it was still down at minus 20, which is pretty cold for this time of year.) Walking has been an exercise I have become faithful to because I enjoy it and because I now understand the benefits of fresh air. Every night at C.H.I.P., we report the time we spent exercising, this is converted to mileage and marked on a map of Canada. We are working our way across the country, starting in Edmonton. Nothing has really changed for me as far as the amount of exercise I do because I am in classes every night!

Tuesday, March 25. C.H.I.P ended last Thursday and we graduate tomorrow night.

We are having a huge banquet (prepared by ourselves).

Friday, March 28, 2003. The C.H.I.P. program wasn't too helpful to me. Many people were having phenomenal results lowering their cholesterol and losing weight but my cholesterol went up and my weight stayed the same. It's a good program for someone who wants to come off the S.A.D. diet (Standard American Diet) but I think more raw food is needed for somebody fighting cancer. My diet for the past year and a half was much more streamlined than what C.H.I.P. teaches.

There are several problems with the program, which make it unsuitable for cancer patients. First of all, the classes were from 7 p.m. to 9:30 p.m., four nights a week. People fighting cancer need rest. They need to be in bed by 9 o'clock. Secondly, there is too much cooked food. Almost all of the recipes were for cooked food, and this produces a more acidic situation in the body tissues. Cancer patients need to eat at least 75 per cent raw in order to kick this bully in the butt. Another problem was the food demos, which were wonderful, were always around 8 p.m. and it is not good to eat in the evening. I think it is a great program, perhaps not the best for me at this time in my life.

So I went all raw today. A banana for breakfast, half a pineapple for lunch and carrot juice for the rest of the day. I am very much in a state of warfare, mentally, physically and spiritually. When a person is attacked the adrenaline kicks in.

Tuesday, April 1, 2003. April Fools Day - it is snowing! I could be in Mexico right now because last week I came so close to booking a flight to Sanoviv. They have a new Medical Review Program where a person can come down for two full days of diagnostics, spa treatment and some of the other therapies available. My oncologist in Edmonton took a full month to write me a prescription for Zoladex, which put me 6 weeks overdue for my injection. I was waiting for him to get approval to have it paid for, but all that time, after several reminders, he still has not applied, so I finally paid for it myself. Whenever I start to feel like I am not being cared for properly, I want to run to Sanoviv where I know I will be looked after. The only thing that stopped me was the cost. Also, I do have resources here that I can use.

The past month I have had a lady staying here who is being treated for esophageal cancer. I have shown her all my motivational videos and I pray that I have been a positive influence in her life. It is a struggle for her to quit smoking but I hope she can find the strength to do it, or ask God for the strength. Without God, I would not have the motivation to continue juicing day after day. I just made up a batch of eight cups to take out to Doug's farm tomorrow. I am going out to help with the calves being born, which I have never experienced before.

One very satisfying thing that happened over the past few weeks was a phone call that I got from a fellow suffering with colon cancer. I was able to put him in touch with Sanoviv and he is going down with his wife in a couple of weeks. I know it will change his life. I have had quite a few calls from people with cancer and have been able to make referrals.

Saturday, April 5, 2003. Well I never actually saw some calves being born, but I got to feed a newborn orphan calf. We mixed up colostrum in a two-litre bottle and fed him in the barn. Then the next day Doug hooked him up with a cow that had lost her calf. It can take a few days for the mother to accept the calf so sometimes they have to put her head in a metal grip while the baby is feeding. It is unbelievably hard work being outside all day, getting in and out of trucks, opening and closing gates, lifting calves and walking around checking things. I am sure most people don't realize the amount labour that goes into producing beef. They work 7 days a week, at least 12 hours a day. I think they need at minimum one day of rest. I was completely exhausted after one day!

Part of my fatigue was due to the fact that my breast has been swollen for a couple of weeks and it takes awhile for the Zoladex to kick in. I guess I still need to conserve my energy to fight the cancer. Just going for walks is all I can do right now, but I sure want to get to the place where I can do more physical work.

Tuesday, April 8, 2003. Last week was freezing winter weather and today was a gorgeous summer day. Even though I was busy at work, I managed to get in a 40-minute walk.

This evening I read about benefits of sunlight that I was unaware of. Sunlight improves blood circulation; increases the amount of blood that is pumped by the heart with each contraction; increases the oxygen-carrying capacity of the blood; helps to regulate the blood pressure toward a normal, healthy level; increases the number of white blood cells and stimulates their ability to destroy both germs and *cancer* cells. It improves liver function, helps the body to eliminate toxic chemicals and environmental pollutants and increases gamma globulin - a protein that helps the body fight infection. As well, it stabilizes blood sugar levels and lowers cholesterol and triglycerides in the blood. Sunlight may decrease cholesterol by more than 33 percent. It converts cholesterol and ergosterol in the skin to vitamin D, but only to safe levels. There is more: sunlight improves muscle tone and endurance; increases body metabolism by stimulating thyroid gland function; enhances mental outlook; lessens stress and promotes healing.[34] No wonder we cannot survive without sunlight! The next time I am out for a walk I am going to visualize those white blood cells destroying any cancer cells that might be hanging around.

Monday, April 14, 2003. My oncologist did eventually apply for coverage for the Zoladex but the director turned down the request again. I really do not want to mention my doctor's name because he confessed to me that he finds it frustrating to work within the confines of a rigid system. Apparently it only costs $380 for the Alberta health care system to pay for a mastectomy and $175 per radiation treatment, so the powers that be have decided that this is more cost effective than paying $500/mo. for hormone therapy. It is cheaper for sure, but what bothers me is that I was never even given the option. If I had not gone to Sanoviv, I would have never heard of this therapy. The pharmacist even told me that he knows hormone therapy works, but the Cancer Board has to think of costs. If they know it works, then why was I told two years ago that the only proven treatment is chemotherapy, surgery and radiation?

In one of Dr. Malkmus' audiotapes *(How to Eliminate Sickness)* he states that if estrogen could be removed from women's bodies, breast cancer could virtually be eliminated. That's exactly what

Zoladex does - removes estrogen from the body. So you can poison the cancer, cut the breast off, and radiate the flesh, but if the cause of the problem is still there, the cancer just comes back. But hey, if the woman dies, the cancer board still saved money by not giving her hormone therapy. The woman is just a statistic to them.

Some women may still chose to have chemotherapy, surgery and radiation, but I think they should at least be told that there are other therapies that work. I have seen pictures of cancer growing back in the scar where the breast used to be and I cannot imagine the discouragement a woman must feel to have her breast cut off only to have the cancer continue to grow. There is a sense of betrayal, and in reality, the woman has been betrayed. She was not given all the facts. This of course applies to any form of cancer in either sex - patients are not being given all the facts.

Wednesday, April 23, 2003. Mom made a beautiful Easter dinner this past weekend and it was nice to see my sister and her family who came up from Calgary.

On Saturday, Ivan and I went for a long walk in the river valley which is finally free of snow. He is a friend I met in the Christian singles group and he's been a real blessing to me. He has fixed my car and my toilet and now he has offered to re-shingle my roof, which should have been done a few years ago. There are many projects around this house that should have been done a few years ago but because of my finances being tied up with health concerns (and lack of energy) they just have not been done. Ivan is the kind of person who just sees what needs to be done and does it. In exchange, I can make healthy food to give him to show my appreciation. I am really in awe of people who can fix things with ease and who have tremendous physical strength. I have been so academic all my life.

Friday, April 25, 2003. Dr. Trethart did an Ion Cleanse on me today. The Ion Cleanse basically pulls toxins out of your lymphatic system using osmosis. There was much less lymphatic clogging in my breast afterwards. Dr. Trethart is a doctor in Edmonton who specializes in Nutritional Medicine. I wish there were more doctors like him around. Dr. Trethart also sold me some DMSA, which chelates mercury out of the body. It cost over $100 so it better get the mercury out! Because it also chelates other heavy metals and removes them, I have to take liquid mineral replacement as well. He told me to do this for 3 months to make sure the mercury gets out of all the tissues in my body. I'm hoping that this will start to alleviate my fibromyalgia symptoms, which continue to plague me.

The last few weeks I have been feeling like I am fighting an uphill battle and I have been sliding down more than I have been going up. That feeling was not getting any better so I booked a flight to Sanoviv for the 16th of May. I am going to do their Medical Review program. It is a new three-day program of extensive diagnostics. I'll also spend a couple of days relaxing in the sun.

Monday, May 5, 2003. Henrietta tested me on the Vega machine last week and I was showing high levels of psychological stress. No sign of cancer. I am glad I am going to Sanoviv just for the psychological aspect. The immune system functions much better when you are relaxed.

I just read about a study by Jane Hightower, an internist at California Pacific Medical Center in San Francisco. She found that 89 per cent of the patients who twice a week or more ate large ocean fish had blood mercury levels either just above or up to ten times higher than the five parts per billion recommended by the Environmental Protection Agency (EPA). Just six ounces of tuna contain as much as 35 micrograms of mercury, close to the 38.5 microgram weekly limit recommended by the National Academy of Sciences and the EPA.[35] "Any given carnivorous fish is packing a few meals' worth of the toxic metal, which has long been known to be lethal to cells in the brain and the nervous, immune, and reproductive systems."[36] Dr. Trethart said that the mercury stays in your brain and other parts of your body, and it is crucial to get it out, so I am glad I am taking DMSA.

Sanoviv Medical Review Program

Friday, May 30, 2003. Going to Sanoviv was definitely the right thing to do. I was very stressed when I left Edmonton and I had a bad flu bug. After a day of relaxing in the sun, using the infrared sauna and the hot and cold pools, my cold was gone and I felt like a weight was lifted off me. There is no doubt in my mind that stress affects a person's ability to fight disease. It is so nice to have other people doing the sprouting, gardening, food prep, laundry, cleaning, shopping etc. I love my garden and my house, but they both are a lot of work because I work full time.

I am still waiting for the medical reports to be sent here from Sanoviv, but basically they did not find anything to indicate active cancer. The Mexican oncologist told me I was fortunate to have had an estrogen positive tumor because that enabled them to treat me without surgery. Only 20 per cent of premenopausal breast tumors are estrogen positive, and if the tumor had not been, Dr. Vazquez would have recommended surgery. I would like to know if any woman with an estrogen receptor negative inflammatory breast cancer has ever survived without surgery.

Saturday, May 31, 2003. The last few weeks have been encouraging to me because I have sold almost 40 copies of my testimonial video. It is 45 minutes long and has volumes of information and resources for anyone dealing with any type of cancer. It is called "Overcoming Breast Cancer". Also, a patient from the office where I work called to tell me she is booked to go to Sanoviv on June 24. It makes me really happy because she's one more person who's going to have her life changed for the better.

Today I am going to a picnic with the Christian singles group.

Sunday, June 1, 2003. At my church, we have small groups and the one I just started going to was interested in seeing my testimonial video. It generated a lot of discussion about the kind of food Christians eat and got a lot of people thinking. I was thankful to Suzanne for asking to see it, because I do not always feel a lot of interest in the church. Sometimes Christians have a tendency to write off any new alternative treatment as "new age" when they do not even understand what it is involved.

I remember when Chiropractors were considered new-age by some Christians and now many church people I know go to Chiropractors.

Tuesday, June 10, 2003. Our Christian singles group did a beautiful hike out at Elk Island National Park on Saturday. It was a perfect day for walking - about 24 degrees Celsius. The group roasted hot dogs and I ate my vegetable sandwich - I felt like I had the better deal by far! On Sunday, I took mom out for her birthday to Doan's Vietnamese Restaurant. Mom had never eaten at a Vietnamese restaurant before and she seemed to like it.

This year I am really becoming involved in my garden. I'm so glad to have enough energy to garden and the plants are starting to look quite nice. The only trouble is my back. The chiropractor has told me to take it easy because he is treating me for facet syndrome in the low back right now. If I do any digging, it has to be on my knees. Shovelling is out.

I sure miss the food at Sanoviv. I am dreaming of establishing a Health Retreat here in Edmonton with a well equipped kitchen for preparing live foods, a fitness room with rebounders, a lecture room for watching videos and having classes, an infrared sauna, a massage room, and everything else that Sanoviv has. God, could it be? There are many people in Edmonton doing such good work in the area of alternative medicine but we need a place where it all comes together. I know I need to permanently live in a healthy environment. I am going to do everything I can to make this house a totally healthy place but it is not big enough to have a health retreat. A lifestyle centre.

Hallelujah Acres has a Total Health Retreat at their headquarters in Shelby, North Carolina and I'm thinking of going there in a few months. I need to get away every so often and this health retreat seems reasonable. It does not offer half of what Sanoviv offers but it does have the raw food. Maybe the more retreats I go to the more ideas I will get of what would be possible in Edmonton.

Monday, June 16, 2003. The last few days have been very active and very beautiful. On Saturday, my friend Jason and I went for a four-hour walk in the river valley. Jason has type-one diabetes. He loves to go walking. It was bright and sunny for the first three hours, then a black cloud came from nowhere and we got drenched! Trying to get shelter under a poplar tree didn't work so we ran back to the truck. On Sunday, we walked for another couple of hours and the sun held out for us.

Today, bright and early, my friend Teresa came over. She was looking for work and I needed some help around the house, so the two needs went together. When I came home from work, there were eight cups of carrot with greens juice in the fridge, the garage was clean, the garden was weeded, the laundry was done and the lawn was mowed. What an unbelievably hard worker Teresa is! I could not have done that much physical work in one day, mostly because of my back. I think she should work at the future health retreat!

Thursday, June 19, 2003. Sometimes I wonder if it is really worth the cost to eat organic, but I recently read a newsletter that assured me it is. Friends that I took a food prep course from put out a news bulletin and they reported on a new study from Seattle that showed pesticide levels to be nine times higher in children eating a conventional diet as opposed to children eating organic food.[37] They also mentioned a report from the Journal of Agricultural and Food Chemistry that shows organically grown foods are higher in cancer- fighting antioxidants than conventional food. "The new study suggests pesticides and herbicides actually thwart the production of phenolics, which act as a plant's natural defence and also are good for human health. Phenolics have potent antioxidant activity and are produced in plants in response to environmental stressors, such as insects or competing plants. The need for these natural safeguards decreases with the use of herbicides and pesticides. This decrease is reflected in the amount of antioxidants the plants produce and that we get in the food. You can read more about this at *www.rense.com/general35/cnn.htm*"[38]

Sunday, June 22, 2003. It is rainy and cold today so I have been reading *The Mad Cowboy*, a book written by a rancher who became a vegetarian. Alberta recently had its first reported case of Mad

Cow disease (Bovine Spongiform Encephalopathy, BSE). This book has been on my list for a while, so I thought now would be a good time to get it. When I talked to my friend Doug, who is a rancher, about this mad cow disease, he said he was not surprised it happened because so many farmers feed their cows ground up animal parts and cows are grass-eaters. This author said the same thing. "Until we stop the transformation of cattle into carnivores, until we can be 100 per cent sure that they are no longer consuming the blood and fecal material of their own species and the meat and bone meal of any other animal, the risks of Mad Cow disease and a consequent human epidemic of CJD will be with us." (p 101)[39]

CJD is Creutzfelt-Jacob Disease and it causes dementia, leaving holes in the brains of its victims. It can occur spontaneously in one in a million people or it can be transmitted by eating an infected animal. There has been an increase in CJD in Britain since their mad cow outbreak in the 1990s and Richard Lacey, a microbiologist, "projects the worst-case scenario at two hundred thousand British deaths annually beginning around the year 2015." (p 97, Mad Cowboy) This is because the estimated incubation time for the disease in humans is thought to be from ten to thirty years. Potentially, there could be an increase in CJD in Canada because it is not known if other cows with BSE were slaughtered and processed into the food chain. The only reason this one was reported is because someone at the slaughterhouse noticed the cow was dropping; the farmer himself did not report it. It is a scary thought for anyone who eats red meat - I am just glad that I am not one of them. There is nothing I can do about what I consumed before becoming a vegan so I will not worry about it!

Sunday, June 29, 2003. This weekend has been totally relaxing. On Friday Jason and I went to see "Bruce Almighty" with Jim Carey. I was not sure what to expect but it was really funny. Jason has also discovered the value of humor therapy in keeping him healthy. We have been doing a lot of walking also. The walking helps keep his diabetes under control and it helps me fight the cancer.

Looking through my reports from Sanoviv, I can see there are many things I have to work on. The live blood analysis showed a few problems, which are ongoing. There is still a proteolytic enzyme deficiency, so I started taking enzymes again. The analysis showed the presence of sialic acid, which I have to look up because I do not know what it is. The red blood cells were slightly stacked, which is due to a pH imbalance and/or an electrolyte imbalance from bad absorption, poor mineral intake, catabolic chemistry or low intensity magnetic fields. I did slack off taking my minerals and antioxidants so I am taking them more often now because of this report. There is still chemical toxicity, grade two out of three, which is to be expected because I am chelating mercury out of my body and taking some medications. As a result of the chemicals, my liver is stressed, so I have to start taking milk thistle again. There are so many things to keep on top of all the time. Undoing the damage of decades of neglect is not easy.

The Diagnostic Functional Medicine test (DFM) showed energy-sapping processes and geopathy, which is caused by the unnatural environment in which we live. Dr. Vazquez told me to throw the electrical equipment and the computer at work away but I do not think my boss would like that! (Some day maybe I can live in paradise) It also showed rheumatic form-cycle, which is basically an arthritic process. The suggested remedy was metabolic therapy, which I have to get clarified.

The Vega test showed cadmium stress, so I have to find out where that could be coming from. It also showed a problem in the ascending colon, which does not surprise me, so I need to continue with colon hydrotherapy. There is still a problem with immune deficiency and carcinosis. The medical dictionary says carcinosis is the condition of having a carcinoma anywhere in the body. We know there are still cancer cells in the breast because every time I take a break from the estrogen blockers my breast flares up.

What I can find out about cadmium from the encylopedia is that it "is a soft, silvery-white metallic element used for alloys and plating. Friedrich Stromeyer of Germany discovered it in 1817. For every ten million parts of the earth's crust, only about five parts are cadmium. The metal occurs with zinc minerals and is obtained as a by-product of zinc refining.

Cadmium is poisonous. People have become seriously ill or have died soon after breathing cadmium dust or fumes of cadmium oxide. Small amounts of cadmium entering the body over long periods may also damage the kidneys and deform bones. As people became concerned about environmental pollution, they feared that hazardous amounts of cadmium were reaching the environment from widespread industrial use of the metal.

Industry uses cadmium in alloys for high-speed bearings, and as a protective coating for other metals. Cadmium is often used instead of zinc for galvanizing iron and steel. Cadmium rods are used in nuclear reactors to control nuclear reactions."[39] I need to find an environmental expert to learn how I could have been exposed to cadmium. Actually, I would like to talk to an environmental expert about many questions I have, and even have my home assessed.

Well, I am starting to feel pretty tired. I soaked up a lot of sun today. It was nice to be in the backyard listening to the chickadees chirping.

Sunday, July 6, 2003. Now I'm wondering if cadmium is used in nuclear medicine to do bone scans and other tests. I will have to make some inquiries with the department of nuclear medicine to find out.

Yesterday we got lots of fresh air. I went walking with Jason and a few other people along the trails by the Sturgeon River, we strolled through the outdoor market, and then in the evening we went to a pig roast. Of course I did not eat any pig but it was very nice to be out in the country.

Sunday, July 13, 2003. There is a place here in Edmonton called Earth's General Store, which has all kinds of information about achieving an environmentally healthy home. I purchased some concentrated acetic acid vinegar for killing dandelions and other weeds. I finally feel I have a safe way to get rid of weeds. I also bought a book called *Prescriptions for a Healthy House.* Reading that book is going to be a journey into a whole new world.

The author says, "according to the EPA (Environmental Protection Agency), of the more than 80,000 chemicals common in commercial use today, fewer than 1,000 have been tested for toxic effects on the human nervous system. The limited testing that has been implemented rarely takes into consideration the ongoing, low-level exposure to hundreds of chemicals we inhale or absorb simultaneously throughout our daily lives."[40] There is information in this book about what to look for in a safe bed and where to get one (Not available in Edmonton at this point). A "chemical mattress" is manufactured primarily with synthetic materials derived from crude oil and natural gas, whereas an organic mattress is made with organic cotton and chemical-free wool. A mattress label will tell you that it is made of, for instance, polyurethane foam, styrofoam, nylon and polyester, but it will not list which chemicals these materials are made from. This means that eight hours a day you are sleeping on chemicals of which you have no idea the effect on your body.

Monday, July 28, 2003. It has been 2 years since I first went to Sanoviv, a very sick puppy. Last weekend I went white-water rafting on the Kananaskis River so I have come a long way!

Does Anybody Understand Hormones?

I've been trying to understand hormones. The reason I'm doing research is because the side effects from the Zoladex are not pleasant and even the doctors do not seem sure about how to can alleviate the symptoms. I stopped the Zoladex again for a month because I was in agony. My joints were so stiff, I had a trigger thumb, my bone density decreased considerably in the past year and a half, and the menopause symptoms were getting to me. I told Dr. Vazquez, I could not take the pain anymore and he said, "What choice do you have?" (meaning do this or have the surgery). I think there are things that could be done to alleviate some of these symptoms, but I have to discover them myself. Dr. Vazquez did sell me estriol cream a year ago and he did not think it would affect the tumor, but he wasn't sure. My oncologist in Edmonton said it would not affect it and Henrietta was quite sure it would. So I use it once in awhile.

Dr. Christiane Northrup's book, *The Wisdom of Menopause* came to my rescue. She has clarified so many things for me. It seems that even doctors do not understand hormones all that well. "The testing method employed by most medical practices is to draw a blood sample and submit it to a commercial laboratory for analysis of FSH [follicle stimulating hormone] and/or LH [leutinizing hormone] levels. This is based on the fact that at menopause and thereafter, a woman's FSH and LH levels rise to their highest ever. But there are problems with this method. First of all, it will tell you nothing about estrogen levels, because FSH is controlled by inhibin, not by estrogen. (This is one of the reasons why estrogen replacement doesn't decrease FSH levels after menopause.) In addition, during the five or ten years of perimenopause - before menstruation ceases for good - FSH and LH levels can fluctuate widely. The ovaries may become inactive for a few days or weeks and then resume production of eggs. It is possible, for example for a woman's FSH levels to reach postmenopausal levels (greater than 30 IU/l while she is still having normal periods. Her LH levels, meanwhile, will remain in the normal premenopausal range. For that reason, a single high FSH/LH level can't be used to determine whether or not a woman is in menopause. Until a woman has had no periods for a year and has FSH/LH levels well within the postmenopausal range-

FSH greater than 30 IU/l and LH greater than 40 IU/l-it is even possible for her to get pregnant."

"Another common blood test analyzes the total amount of estrogen, progesterone, and or testosterone in the bloodstream. The largest drawback to this method is that most of the hormone so measured is inactive. Thus the standard blood test, which does not distinguish bound from free hormone, will give an irrelevant result, because it measures primarily inactive, unusable, protein-bound hormone.

There are two less common but more useful tests. The costs are equivalent, the ease of drawing the samples is the same or better, the laboratory service is readily available, and studies show that the results provide a very accurate picture of where in the perimenopausal transition a woman's body currently stands. Salivary hormone testing measures the free hormone present in the saliva, which has been shown to be comparable to what is present in other body tissues. Saliva does not contain measurable levels of protein-bound (inactivated) hormone. Used until recently primarily in research, salivary hormone testing is a technology that has proven reliable for roughly thirty years but is still unfamiliar to many practicing physicians. Blood tests for free (unbound) hormone levels are another viable choice." (p 114)[41]

Now that I know what the LH/FSH levels are supposed to be, I can request my blood work results and actually understand what they mean. Dr. Northrup explains everything so clearly. It's so crucial that I understand estrogen because my tumor is fueled by this hormone. "Estrogen actually encompasses three distinct estrogenic compounds produced naturally in the body: estradiol, estrone, and estriol. Estriol reaches its highest level during pregnancy; it has weaker biological effects on breast and uterine tissue than do estrone and estradiol. (Women with naturally higher estriol levels appear to have lower breast cancer rates than other, which has led some practitioners to prescribe estriol to decrease the risk of breast cancer. Much more research is needed to establish the effectiveness of this approach.)" (p143) Knowing this, I feel much more relaxed using estriol cream.

Estrogen dominance is another thing she explains that I had never heard about before. Apparently, in the perimenopausal years estrogen can become dominant and progesterone can decline. "Because the body is designed for progesterone and estrogen to be present in a dynamic counterbalance with each other, the result is estrogen dominance, with symptoms of both progesterone deficiency and relative estrogen excess." (p 146)[41] Dr. Northrup states that there is a growing body of evidence that points to estrogen dominance as a major factor in promoting breast or uterine cancer in susceptible women. The symptoms of estrogen excess are: bilateral pounding headache, recurrent vaginal yeast infections, breast swelling and tenderness, depression, nausea, vomiting, bloating, leg cramps, yellow-tinged skin, and excessive vaginal bleeding. I mostly had the breast swelling, tenderness, bloating and depression before I was diagnosed with cancer.

Bone density is a big concern being on Zoladex. According to the World Health Organization (WHO), if a reading is less than -2.5, the patient has osteoporosis, but the National Osteoporosis Foundation (NOF) says less than -2.0 is osteoporosis. My last reading at Sanoviv was -2.1 so I really need to do something. I e-mailed Dr. Vaszquez and asked his opinion about how I can treat the osteoporosis because it was never discussed when I was down there. All the focus was on treating the cancer which of course is the life-threatening issue. He recommended ipriflavone from the health food store and/or aridia, which is an extremely expensive IV infusion prescribed by the doctor. My doctor here is not familiar with prescribing aridia so I'll go with the ipriflavone for now.

Dr. Northrup mentions a urine test for bone breakdown products, which can give a reading of the metabolic state of the bones long before a bone density test will register a problem. It also gives a way to monitor progress once treatment is initiated. So I have to ask about that too. I know that I have to take responsibility for my bone density because nobody else is.

Thursday, August 21, 2003. I am still studying Dr. Northrup's book. In the chapter on breast health she talks about flaxseed. "Research has shown that women who excrete the highest amount of lignans - which are formed in the intestinal tract from plant materials - have the lowest risk for getting breast cancer. The food source with the highest known concentration of health-promoting lignans is flaxseed. I suggest that you consume ¼ cup of freshly ground flaxseed daily. Diets high in plant materials also tend to be higher in fiber, which has been shown to help the body excrete excess estrogens in the stool." (p 421) Now that I've written this I am going to eat my flaxseed!

Shannon, the student who is staying with me, came back from Saskatchewan this week and brought with her corn and potatoes. We had a corn roast tonight on my new fire pit. I have got piles of sticks and logs from cleaning up overgrowth and dead branches, so I asked Jason to help me build a fire pit last weekend. I should have done it years ago!

Back to Christine Northrup's book. One of the things that I was curious about was whether or not I could take progesterone, because I have a progesterone and estrogen positive tumor. Dr. Northrup answers the question beautifully. "One of the questions I'm frequently asked is whether a woman whose breast cancer has tested positive for progesterone receptors can safely take progesterone. There is a great deal of confusion about what it means to have a breast biopsy that shows that the tumor is positive for progesterone receptors, especially in those women who have been using bioidentical progesterone at the time of the diagnosis.

Here are the facts. All breast cancers that are positive for progesterone receptors are also estrogen receptor-positive. Because estrogen is known to stimulate growth of these types of cancer cells, many people automatically assume that progesterone must do the same. Just the opposite is true. Positive progesterone receptors indicate that a cancer is receptive to the balancing and anti-cancer effects of progesterone.

To understand this apparent paradox, remember that hormones in the bloodstream and the fluid surrounding cells work by uniting with receptors on the surface of the cell. The hormone fits the receptor like a key in a lock. If the right receptor is there, the hormone message makes its way to the chromosomes and turns on the appropriate gene to produce a specific cellular effect. Progesterone signals the cell to stop multiplying, while estrogen signals the opposite. For that reason, bioidentical progesterone is probably beneficial for women with progesterone receptor-positive breast cancer.

While I'm convinced that bioidentical progesterone is safe and even beneficial for women with estrogen and progesterone positive beast cancers, this is a controversial area. Use your inner guidance and consult with your doctor." (p 441 - 443) I did consult with my doctor and he told me absolutely not to use it so I have to pray about it. No wonder hormones are so confusing to lay people - doctors don't even agree about how to use and balance them!

Saturday, August 23, 2003. It's starting to feel like fall outside. I just got back from the Corn Maze, which is an amazing place. Just outside of Edmonton, a farmer has put pathways all through his corn field. People form a team and together the team follow a list of clues to make the way through the maze. It is a fun way to go for a walk with friends and get fresh air. Sherree organized that activity - she has a real talent for organizing fun things.

Thursday, September 4, 2003. My breast became inflamed after using estriol cream for a week so I quit using it. My take on it is that estrogen positive breast cancer does react to estriol cream and I'm staying away from it.

Saturday, September 13, 2003. We're having a really nice autumn. The tomatoes are still on the vine. Usually they are frosted out by now. Several people have given Shannon and I apples so we have been making "apple pie" smoothies. I got the recipe from the Hallelujah Acres newsletter. It's one cup of fresh apple juice, one frozen banana, three dates and one half teaspoon of cinnamon blended in the blender.

Since it's such a beautiful day a few of us are going walking in Dawson Park this afternoon.

Wednesday, September 17, 2003. When I saw Dr. Trethart several months ago he recommended a product called Thymucin and a book called *Your Body Doesn't Lie*. I finally got around to buying it and now I understand why he wants me on Thymucin. The book explains that the thymus actually plays an important role in the body, but when there is stress the thymus cannot function at optimal capacity, if at all. Lymphocytes actually come to the thymus and mature there, then the lymphocytes go to the lymph nodes and the spleen where they give rise to T cells (T for thymus). The T cells then do their work of scouting out cancer cells and infectious agents. Thymus hormones go through the blood stream and continue to exert an influence over the T cells. If there is stress the thymus can shrink to half its normal size in 24 hours. With all the stress I've had my thymus must have been shrivelled to nothing before I got cancer. The author of this book sites examples of cancer and pneumonia being turned around after thymus extract was injected (p39).[42] Current medical practices pay no attention whatsoever to the thymus gland or the lymphatic system as a whole. Certainly nobody until Dr. Trethart has ever mentioned it to me.

Hallelujah Acres

Tuesday, October 7, 2003. I am so encouraged! I just spent four days down at Hallelujah Acres Total Health Retreat. This health centre does a few tests that I did not have at Sanoviv. For example, I had an iridology exam, which is an examination of the iris of the eye. The doctor who examined me found a few things wrong: my colon has minute pockets or diverticuli, I have a malabsorption problem, my lymphatic system is stressed, and I have markings above the pupil indicative of chronic stress or chronic pain. There was weakness in my ovaries. He did not see any sign of cancer! (I just got my breast MRI results today and it also showed no sign of cancer). I'm impressed that the iridology exam shows the same results that all the other testing reveals.

I was not going to have colon therapy at Hallelujah Acres because I can get it here in Edmonton, but then I took a look at the equipment Health Retreat and changed my mind. I had never seen anything like it and being the curious person that I am, I had to try it. The therapist had what is called an "open system" as opposed to the old style "closed system". The speculum that is inserted into the rectum is much smaller and easier to take and the flow and release is more controlled by the patient. I was able to get the ascending colon cleansed which has not always been possible in the past. A lot of lymphatic debris and mucus debris was released. (I realize that probably only people fighting serious disease are actually going to be interested in reading this!) The reason this is so crucial is that when the colon is not eliminating old lymph, it becomes backed-up in the rest of the body and that is a huge problem with cancer.

Dr. Norman Walker taught that different areas of the colon are related to various parts of the body. He has a famous chart with the entire colon mapped out. For example, if there is impaction or excessive fermentation in the part of the ascending colon corresponding to the mammary glands, "it is more than likely that the lymph glands in the area of the breast may collect waste matter, probably from the colon, and store it in the lymph glands of the breast, causing a lump to appear - as a warning. I have known such cases where the application of colon irrigations caused the lumps to disappear within a matter of days. The most important warnings of neglecting the colon are glandular disturbances." (p22)[43] Now that might sound kind of far-fetched, except that every time I have had a colonic and we have managed to get the water around to the ascending colon, my breast is much less lumpy afterward. So I am totally convinced that Dr. Walker is right. (The fact that he lived to 118 years shows that he had a few things about the body figured out!) The Hallelujah Acres Health store has a whole rack devoted to Dr. Walker's books.

Saturday, October 11, 2003. Hallelujah Acres puts a huge emphasis on eliminating the "Five Deadly Whites" which are animal products, refined flour, sugar, salt and caffeine. This is the same teaching as Sanoviv and all the other raw food teachers I have encountered. For breakfast, they recommend a teaspoon of Barley Green mixed with four to five ounces of water and a cup of carrot juice. No solid food is consumed until lunch time. The reason for this is Dr. Malkmus believes the colon needs a rest from constant digestion. I have been taking Barley Green for breakfast all week and I like it. It is not a huge change for me because I was just having fruit for breakfast before. Hallelujah Acres cautions cancer patients against having a lot of fruit because of the high sugar content. High vegetable, moderate fruit intake was also what Sanoviv recommended.

One of the highlights of the retreat was hearing Dr. Malkmus speak. He did his *How to Eliminate Sickness* lecture on Saturday, October 4. He has been doing this talk on the first Saturday of the month for years. He is energetic and full of passion for what God has led him to do. One of the things he said that stood out was that since he started the raw food diet at the age of 42 years, his eye glass prescription got progressively weaker until he no longer needed glasses! He is going to be 70 and his vision is perfect!

There are a few tips about juicing that I learned at the retreat, which have caused me to adjust my juicing regimen. The first one is that juice made in the champion juicer is only good for 8 hours. It has to be made in the morning and drunk throughout the day. Juice made in a green star juicer can last from 24 to 48 hours depending on how it is stored. Hallulujah Acres has had the juices tested and these were the results. Now I make the juice in the morning and take it to work with me. Two years ago, I could not have done this as I usually crawled out of bed five minutes before I went to work, still groggy from antidepressant medication. Then I needed a cup of coffee to wake myself up.

Tuesday, October 14. I received a wonderful gift at Hallelujah Acres. One of the ladies gave me a copy of *Recipes for Life* by Rhonda Malkmus. While it is a recipe book, the first part of the book is full of information about food. I have known for two years that we get more than enough protein from vegetables and fruits, but I did not know that some of them actually contain all eight essential amino acids. (Our bodies are able to produce 15 amino acids, but eight need to be obtained from food making a total of 23. The eight that we get from food are called "essential" amino acids. "There are many vegetables and some fruits that contain all eight essential amino acids including carrots, brussel sprouts, cabbage, cauliflower, corn, cucumbers, eggplant, kale, okra, peas, potatoes, summer squash, sweet potatoes, tomatoes and bananas."[44] God is truly amazing. The diet that He provided for us in Genesis 1:29 has everything that we need. I'm just concerned that most of our society believes the myth we have been taught that protein must be obtained from meat.

Wednesday, October 15, 2003. Now that the weather is getting cold again, it is a huge challenge not to eat a lot of cooked food. To stay on the Hallelujah diet I need to eat a large salad for lunch and a large salad for supper plus a little bit of cooked food after the evening salad. In this climate a person wants hot food, but when I read about what it does to the human body it makes me want to take it in limited quantities. "During the 1930s a study was conducted which showed that when cooked food is eaten, the white blood cells have to stop their work protecting the body and must help with the digestion of the non-food poisons that have entered the system. When the same foods were eaten in their raw state, there was no change in the blood chemistry." (p80)[45] Becoming vegan was not that hard for me, but being a raw food vegan is much more of a challenge. Since we have a limited number of enzymes, it is only wise to eat raw foods, which still have their enzymes intact.

Sunday, October 26, 2003. Yesterday Irma, my Seventh Day Adventist friend, and I drove out to Lavoy to visit Rudy and Jeannie and her parents at the Abundant Life Therapy Centre. It's been eight months since I last saw them. I think they were really glad to see two people who have been through their cleanse program and who are sticking to the vegan diet. We had lunch with Bud and Donna, Jeannie's parents, and then had devotions with Rudy and the five patients who are going through the 10 day cleanse right now. They asked me to share my testimony, especially to encourage one of the ladies there who has cancer. It is beautiful to see how these two couples are transforming that old run-down Lavoy Hotel into a vibrant health work for the Lord.

At Abundant Life, guests eat a big breakfast with lots of raw fruit and then at about 2 o'clock they have a big lunch with lots of raw vegetables and a bit of cooked rice or potato, then no more food for the rest of the day. At Hallelujah Acres, they have no solid food until about noon when they have a large raw salad, and then another raw salad at supper. At both places, people are only eating two meals a day, it's just that one eliminates breakfast and the other eliminates supper. Dr. Lorraine Day has three meals a day. I have not completely decided on which way to go, but I do like having a bit of fruit at breakfast and something warm like a baked potato for supper. At least we all agree on the large raw salad at lunch and the vegan menu. I think the main thing is to eat vegan and mostly raw because all three of these teachers are getting excellent results with only minor variations in their programs.

Last week, I helped Jason make a lentil loaf. For him to ask for help making a lentil loaf is a huge step because he has been eating hamburger for supper all his life. Being at Hallelujah Acres was really good for him and he has started telling many people about the Hallelujah diet.

Tuesday, November 4, 2003. Yesterday I had a couple of friends over. I made them some recipes from Rhonda Malkmus' book. I have wanted to try Baba Ganoush for a long time and Rhonda has a good recipe for that. It's a spread made with eggplant, lemon, garlic and tahini. My boss took the day off so I had a whole day to create new dishes. I would love to do that more often but right now God has me in this job.

The walking group that I started on Saturdays is really taking off. I thought with winter coming that participation would taper off but we had eight people out last week. After one and one half hours, we were all sweating, even though it was below zero.

The new Sanoviv website went up last week. They have wonderful testimonials on it, and mine is one of them!

Friday, November 14, 2003. "The *length of life* is inversely proportional to the *rate* of exhaustion of the enzyme potential of an organism. The increased use of food enzymes promotes a *decreased rate* of exhaustion of the enzyme potential."[45] That is the enzyme nutrition axiom by Dr. Edward Howell. The importance of enzymes is really stressed at Hallelujah Acres. Most of us in North America deplete our enzyme supply by eating a lot of cooked, dead food. I was told at the Total Health Retreat and at Sanoviv to have enzymes with every meal so I'm not using up so much of my enzyme potential. There are three main types of enzymes: metabolic, digestive and food (raw, living food). If you're not consuming food with the enzymes still intact then your body is forced to use up its reserves, depleting your life force. Enzyme under-nutrition is one of the biggest causes of the deadly diseases. So a person can eat good food, but if it's all cooked, that person will be malnourished.

Monday, November 17, 2003. "It is decidedly unbecoming for those possessing the tools of science to close their eyes to the possibility that those diseases, which are human trademarks, such as cancer and heart disease, are the products of disturbed metabolism induced partly by the hidden machinations of food enzyme deficiency."[45] I'm finding out that there's a controversy about enzymes in the scientific world. The official position of chemistry, which has been taught for almost a century, is that enzymes are not used up in the process of doing their work. What Dr. Edward Howell and many others are contending is that they are used up, and once they are gone the life force departs from a person. If there are no more metabolic enzymes the body organs simply cannot function.

Dr. Howell has much to say about lipase and fat digestion. Because the fats we eat are generally separated from their enzymes by refining and cooking, we are unable to digest them until they get to the intestines and even then, with difficulty. If the fats were raw and unrefined, digestion could begin in the upper stomach because they would still have the lipase intact. "When fat is eaten raw, with its lipase undamaged by heat, it can be digested along with protein and carbohydrate in the upper (food-enzyme) stomach prior to the time the acidity becomes strong enough to prevent further action."[45] This worked for the Eskimos, who ate huge amounts of raw blubber and had low cholesterol. (Not that we need raw fat, it's the lipase we need) It seems to me, that with all the problems we have with cholesterol these days, Dr. Howell's book should be required reading in all the medical schools. I guess it's easier just to give people medication. Should we be surprised that it is not among the medical school textbooks?

Saturday, November 22, 2003. It's -27° Celsius with the wind chill and we still had 4 people out for the walk today!

Wednesday, December 10, 2003. The last two Saturdays 11 people have participated in the river valley walk. It's neat to see how this walking group is gathering momentum.

Tuesday, December 16, 2003. All this reading about enzymes led me to purchase a huge container of enzymes from Aveena. I have two friends who come walking with me who are really on the same wavelength as me as far as health and they invited me to a lecture by Michael O'Brien. I was very impressed by his talk, because it confirmed everything I have learned thus far. I am now taking five capsules with every meal and five capsules in between meals. This is a progressive learning curve. I first learned about enzymes at Sanoviv and I would take them once in awhile, then I learned more at Hallelujah Acres and started to take enzymes more often, now I am totally convinced that enzymes are vital to maintaining health. I make sure they are part of my meals. The more something is reinforced, the more it sinks in. It is interesting that I met Ted and Diane around the same time I went to Hallelujah Acres.

I thanked Dr. Trethart for putting me on the DMSA. When I told him that my fibromyalgia cleared up after 15 years of being on medications, Dr. Trethart was really happy. He surprised me though. He told me I should do another three months of it to clear up any residual heavy metal toxicity that could be disturbing the breast tissue. I take one capsule in the morning and a tablespoon of liquid minerals at night to replace any of the good metals that get chelated out with the mercury.

Dr. Trethart is also helping me with my bone density problem and my cholesterol problem. He put me on strontium and high dose vitamin D for the bones. The strontium surprised me because it is not something that you usually hear recommended for bone density problems. In 1959, the Mayo clinic did a study on strontium and osteoporosis and got good results. Strontium is in the same mineral family as calcium and magnesium. Dr. Trethart gave me an article on it and the author wonders why things died down in the strontium/osteoporosis world after such a wonderful study was published. He speculates "the patent medicine industry tried its best to come up with a synthetic version of strontium that they could trademark and make a profit from. But when they couldn't find one, they gave up. Unpatentable substances just aren't researched by patent medication companies, which pretend to be interested in your health but really are only interested in you if they can sell you a patent medication."[46] This author says it doesn't matter if it's strontium ranelate, strontium gluconate, strontium lactate or strontium carbonate, as long as it's strontium, it's good for you! Strontium can be found in spices, seafood, whole grains, root and leafy vegetables, and legumes, but not in quantities large enough to have an effect if you already have osteoporosis.

I've Survived Three Years Without Surgery!

Thursday, January 1, 2004. I brought in the New Year in a wonderful way. I was at a party at the Alliance Church out in Fort Saskatchewan, Alberta. After the party, my old friend Lorri, whom I haven't seen for a year, invited me to stay overnight at her home so I wouldn't have to drive back in the snow storm. It was great to catch up with her. We used to spend hours together hiking, camping and talking, before LorrI went up north to work as a nurse for many years. Fort Saskatchewan is still a ways to come into the city. I know I shouldn't have stayed up so late, but it's only once a year!

Christmas was in Mexico this year! Allison wanted to get away from the commercialism of the season. I don't think the spending and gorging ones' self with food has much to do with celebrating Jesus anyways so when Allison asked me to join her in Mexico I said "great idea!" We stayed in an all-inclusive resort in Puerto Vallarta. Bicycles were free, along with water aerobics, stretching classes and three meals. Not eating organic food for a whole week concerned me, but I stuck to fresh fruits for breakfast and vegetables for lunch and supper. Not having carrot juice for a whole week *really* concerned me, but I did find a juice place on the second day and was able to buy a litre there. Now that I'm back home and making eight cups a day again, I notice that my breast is much less lumpy, so when I don't take my "medicine" my body lets me know! The lady at the juice shop in Puerto Vallarta told me that people like to buy the carrot juice because of the nice color tan it gives them. (Just an added bonus for eating the way God wants us to!)

Thursday, January 15, 2004. I deeply feel my need for God. I crave His presence. Last night at church, when we sang the song *Amazing Love* I wept. I feel I cannot do a thing without Him. Dina lent me a book called *Listening Prayer.* The author talks about our deep need to pursue a personal relationship with Christ. "We need spiritually dense foods. We can gorge ourselves on bible study, prayer, Christian Fellowship, praise and worship, witnessing and faithful church attendance, but still lack a missing nutrient. What or Who is it? The missing part is God Himself. It takes a personal experience and a close friendship with God to produce in us the perfect state of spiritual health, regardless of what else we eat or do not eat in the way of spiritual food. Without this personal relationship, we are helpless to digest and assimilate the spiritual diet that will produce the proper results within us."[47] God I need You, desperately.

Thursday, January 22, 2004. Next month it will be 3 years since I was diagnosed. Far from being dead, I seem to be very much on the go! I'm walking every day, playing volleyball on the weekends, and working full time, but what I really love is working as a consultant for Sanoviv. On a regular basis, I talk with people who are disillusioned with the medical system and are looking for alternatives.

One of the girls I walk with, lent me a book called *My God I Thought You'd Died* by Claude Dosdall. I thought the title was funny. He had a malignant brain tumor, did a lot of work on himself and overcame it. We have a lot of education to do before people understand that cancer is only something that can bully you to death if you let it. With faith, the right information, and obedience to make the lifestyle change, the bully can be silenced.

Sunday, January 25, 2004. Claude Dosdall speaks about finding the meaning of your cancer. This is difficult work. It continues to be painful for me to look at all the things that happened that contributed to this disease. I am determined to rise above every negative thing with the help of God. I believe this started as far back as when I was a teenager. The severe depression that I went into after I was assaulted really suppressed my immune system and set up the conditions for cancer to grow. Depression and despair affect the limbic system in the brain, which sends a message to the hypothalamus. This in turn affects the immune system and the endocrine system. The immune activity decreases and abnormal cells increase. This is the message of Carl Simonton, from his psycho-physiological model of cancer growth.

Wednesday, February 4, 2004. Earlier this week, I visited a lady who is the sister of a friend at church. She has gone through the prescribed treatments of the cancer institute and now her cancer has returned. The medical establishment has given up on her.

I told her my story, and to make a long story short, she's on her way to Sanoviv at the end of the week!

Monday, February 9, 2004. Yesterday was our monthly potluck for the Vegetarian Association of Alberta. They asked me to speak at next month's meeting!

Tuesday, February 17, 2004. Went to a dance on Saturday for the first time in decades! I danced with some nice gentlemen and they patiently tried to teach me. Actually some of them are just learning too so I didn't feel so bad! I play volleyball with a lot of these people so we're all becoming friends.

Today a medical student came to observe our lab and it turned out that she's a seventh day adventist. We had a good talk about preventive medicine and her church.

Tuesday, March 9, 2004. I spent my 3rd year "victory over cancer" anniversary down at Sanoviv. I felt a very deep sense of relaxation while I was there, especially during the Vega therapies. A friend of mine, Arlene, went down with me and she really had her eyes opened. Wheat grass, colon therapy, green juice, yoga, raw food - all new things for her! There were quite a few other women down there with breast cancer and we've formed an e-mail support group. A couple of them had gone the route of mastectomy and their cancer had spread to other parts of their bodies. The sense of urgency that I have to get this book to press grows stronger every time I hear a story like that. One of the biggest enemies people have is fear. One little lump can get a woman so terrified that she'll have both her breasts off. Without being told anything about boosting the immune system, and how fear can affect the immune system, the person allows cancer, the bully, to have power over her.

Thursday, March 11,2004. I just did my rebounding and while I was jumping up and down I was thinking about how happy I was making my lymphocytes. I've been reading *The Cancer Answer* by Albert Carter and he teaches, in a very creative way, how to boost your immune system. Throughout the book he has a conversation with "Larry", his lymphocyte, and Larry tells him what he needs in order to best do his job as a killer T cell. Rebounding uses the forces of acceleration and deceleration, as well as the forces of gravity, which subjects all the cells in the body to an increased G-force. This makes all the cells stronger. If there is no gravity the cells become less active, as documented in a scientific study of U.S. astronauts and Russian cosmonauts. Einstein said in 1911 that the forces of acceleration and deceleration have the same effect on the human body as gravity does. This is what makes rebounding the perfect exercise.[48]

"Larry Lymphocyte" also says that beta-carotene destroys the mucus layer around a cancer cell making it easier for him (Larry) to do his job.(p228) That gives me another positive thing to visualize when I'm drinking carrot juice!

Monday, March 22, 2004. My friend Sharon in Hay River sent an email last week about a dream she had of me. The message in the dream was that the Lord was going to use me to heal women who were broken-hearted and that I would be totally and completely healed. In her dream the Lord was speaking to me and saying that I had been wounded in the past but I would be restored. He had never intended for those things to happen to me, but everything would work out for good in the future. The message was repeated three times. I was very encouraged by that!

Wednesday, March 24,2004. Last night I was talking to a lady with breast cancer and she had been told by a nutritionist at an alternative medical institute that it was not good to drink carrot juice. When I hear that I can't believe the lies that get spread around. Here is what Dr. Norman Walker (remember, the guy who lived to be 119!) has to say about it: "Carrot juice is one of the most healthy and complete foods which the human body can obtain. There is no deleterious effect from drinking quantities of carrot juice. I personally, have consumed ONE GALLON of carrot juice daily, when I felt the need with most beneficial results. To this very day I drink all the carrot juice (plus other vegetable juices that I have the time and the inclination to drink. *Don't let anybody tell you that fresh raw carrot and other vegetable juices are anything BUT healthy and helpful."* [49] Thank you Dr. Walker!!!

Friday, April 30, 2004. The last ten days I was out at Lavoy, at the Abundant Life Therapy Centre, doing the same cleanse I did last year. There were 7 of us going through the program. We had wheatgrass almost every day. This is not a big flavor favorite with me but the results I got were phenomenal! Wheatgrass has 11 times the calcium of cow's milk, 5 times the iron of spinach, 4 times the vitamin B1 of whole wheat flour, 7 times the vitamin C in oranges and an abundance of vitamin B12. One ounce of wheatgrass has the same nutritional value as 2½ pounds of greens! I had some swollen lymph nodes when I arrived - I knew my immune system was struggling - but by the end of the cleanse they were clear. This was a result of not just the wheatgrass, but the whole program. We got lots of rest, fresh air, sunlight, and detoxification through the drinks, raw food, exercise and the steam baths.

Sunday, May 2, 2004. In Lavoy, Rudy gave me another clue as to why excess estrogen (estrogen dominance) can occur in women. When the liver becomes congested it prevents glucuronic acid from being formed, and glucuronic acid is what helps to keep estrogen levels down. Before I was diagnosed, my estrogen levels were soaring and my liver was congested from all the medication and animal products I was consuming. I haven't needed to take estrogen blockers for over 2 months now, so I think the estrogen is now at a safe level. Thank you God for leading me down the way I should go!

One of the ladies I know with breast cancer past away today. She had cancer for almost three years before she started to learn about God's ten step health plan. By the time she heard about it, the cancer was in her sternum and she wasn't able to change her habits fast enough to overcome the disease process. This makes me so sad. If she had been sent to the Abundant Life Therapy Centre or a similar institution when she was first diagnosed, and implemented what she was learning, we would be seeing a whole different picture today.

They are able to test cell pH in Lavoy now. To review what I learned, cancer cannot exist in a cell pH of 5.8 or higher.

In ultimate health, saliva pH should be between 7 and 8 and urine will be between 6.8 and 8. Most people do not have this high of a reading. It can take up to three years to restore health if you follow the health plan and eat alkaline foods (raw vegetables and fruits). To test the pH we used color-graded paper with a range between 5 and 8, delineated in increments of point two. Before going to bed we put the paper within arms reach so we did not have to sit up before testing the saliva in the morning. Sitting up causes the digestive juices to flow into the mouth and makes the saliva more alkaline than it normally is. Also it's important to have 5 hours of uninterrupted rest before testing. For example, if you get up to go to the bathroom at 1 a.m. you can't test until 6 a.m. We just had to moisten a little strip of the paper and compare it to the color chart. My saliva was 5.8 before I sat up and 6 after I sat up. My urine was 6. So the good news is that I'm out of the range of cancer and the bad news is that I'm still not in optimal health.

There was one video that we watched that had a huge influence on me, and that was Victoria Butenko. I don't know if the video was called Twelve Steps to Raw Food but she has written a book by that title. After listening to her testimony, I decided to go all raw. After I made that decision, I dropped 4 pounds and I'm continuing to lose. What I've found is that eating cooked food makes me want more cooked food and that's why I'm not losing weight. She talks about how cooked food is an addiction on four levels: chemical, emotional, spiritual and physical. When we eat raw food we are getting the nutrients we need so we don't consume such huge quantities. It is shocking to learn how many gallons of digestive juices are used up when you eat cooked or non-vegan food - two and one half gallons per day! If you eat raw meals your digestive juices drop to 1 cup per day! This is because all the food enzymes are still alive and the body doesn't have to use up its reserves. This is amazing information!

Tuesday, May 25, 2004. For the last couple of weeks I have had company. Most of my free time has been spent going for walks with Barb and Paul and catching up with what's happening in each other's lives. It's been a great blessing! Barbie and I have been friends since University and she led me to the Lord 28 years ago. Since they have been here, we have been going over to Organic Roots a lot to eat and buy groceries. Barbie and her husband Paul are now totally sold on sprouting and bought a huge supply of sprouting seeds to take back up to the Northwest Territories. Now they understand much better the rational behind the approach I am taking to my cancer treatment, after experiencing it firsthand.

Recently I rechecked my pH levels: the urine has gone up to 7.4 and the saliva is about 6.5! That is after just one month of eating all raw! This is amazing! I've known for three years that people get amazing results when they eat all raw and it has taken me this long to put it into practice!

I'm having a big celebration for my 50th birthday! It's coming up in another week!

Wednesday, June 2, 2004. I was very blessed on my birthday. About 50 people were there! My mom did an awesome job of hospitality, as usual. The room was beautifully decorated and she made a display board with pictures from various stages of my life.

Rudy, from Lavoy, sang a song that he wrote called "Praying Child" and he shared a bit about the work they are doing in Lavoy. François, my cousin Janice's husband, told me the evening was a real testimonial to how faith in God can turn a situation around.

Epilogue

Friday, August 20, 2004. I've just returned from Owen Sound, Ontario where I took training at Hallelujah Acres to become a *Back to the Garden* Health Minister. I learned how to run a support group for people who want to live a healthier lifestyle. I'm also qualified to teach the *Get Healthy, Stay Balanced* Course that Hallelujah Acres offers. My first support group will be this Saturday evening! So far there are four people coming, which is about all my living room will comfortably hold!

Tuesday, August 31, 2004. The support group was really successful! Irma was so excited about the *Hallelujah Food Show* videos that she bought the whole set. We had to keep stopping the *Eating in the Outdoors* video, so we could write down the recipes. Irma is planning on making them for her family get together this weekend! I have probably watched the *Eating in the Outdoors* video about 9 times already, because it has so many good recipes. So far I have tried the dehydrated potato chips, the coconut pudding, and the coleslaw with almond mayonnaise. They're all very good.

It was very exciting for me to find out I could eat potato chips and they are actually healthy!

I talked to my mom on the phone tonight. She is using the Barley Max (dehydrated barley juice) from Hallelujah Acres that I gave her! She still comes faithfully and helps me with juicing once a week.

Friday, September 3, 2004. When I look back three and a half years at how I was searching everywhere for answers, I see that many things have been sorted out. I no longer believe that there are different diets for every blood type. I believe that the vegan diet is best for all blood types. Horses have 14 blood types and they all eat the same thing!

Monday, September 5, 2004. The other day I was visiting a woman with Leukemia. She had suffered terrible emotional trauma from a very young age. We had a very long talk and both felt better afterwards. She lent me a book called *Cancer Traditional and New Concepts*. While reading it today, I found an interesting quote: "According to the world famous cancer research physician, Dr. Hans Nieper of Germany: "In Germany it is a law. When someone has cancer, doctors must tell the patient that there are four alternatives: surgery, radiation, chemotherapy or nutrition. The doctor must explain nutrition to the patient, and the patient may take the choice."[50] Oh, what a long way we have to go in Canada! Will the science of raw food nutrition ever be taught to doctors?

Also in the book, *Cancer Traditional and New Concepts*, the author mentions the Hunzas. "In the Himalayan Mountains of Pakistan lives an isolated tribe of people. They live in a beautiful valley called Hunzaland. Travellers reported that the Hunzakuts are very healthy... These peoples' diet consisted of lots of apricots, vegetables, millet and other grains. After Dr. Banik and Renee Taylor published their book on the Hunzaland we all started eating dried apricots... The next explorers also found that they cracked the seeds of the apricots... Apricot kernels have B17".

Until a couple of months ago, I did not know that apricot seeds could be cracked open. Today I hammered some open, and there is a kernel inside that tastes somewhat like bitter almond. Some of them took a fair bit of hammering to get open! Commercially, B17 is called laetrile. Laetrile is known to destroy cancer cells. It is very expensive to purchase laetrile in concentrated form, but it is available in the kernels and seeds of apples, apricots, cherries, nectarines, peaches, pears, plums, prunes, and bitter almonds. It is also found in sprouted lentils, sprouted mung beans, broad beans, chick peas, scarlet runner and Rangoon beans. Almost all wild berries contain laetrile. Chia, flax, sesame and clover seeds have vitamin B17. The grains oat groats, barley, brown rice, buckwheat groats, chia, flax, millet, rye, and wheat berries all have laetrile. It is found in abundance in nature! All of these years I've been throwing away the apricot kernels.

Wednesday, September 8, 2004. The research on hormones continues. I'm finding considerable information on progesterone. Several studies have shown that both "progesterone and synthetic progestins have been found not only to slow bone loss but to increase bone density, as progesterone is a bone-trophic hormone.

Thus, addition of progesterone should be considered when designing a program for osteoporosis prevention."[51] Many authors consider it safe to use on breast cancer patients because it occupies the same receptors that estrogen would also occupy. Estrogen is what causes the breast tissue to grow, but progesterone does not, so you want progesterone in those receptors. Hallelujah Acres has a natural progesterone cream that you can put on your skin and it is well absorbed, so I've been using that. Hallelujah Acres has also produced an audiotape by author John R. Lee which promotes the use of progesterone to deal with menopausal symptoms and bone loss.

Friday, September 10, 1004. Tomorrow we are having a new person join our support group. She really wants to make some improvements in her health. I'm excited!

I don't know exactly where this journey will lead. I'm taking the Lord's hand and going where He tells me to go each day. I know that I will be sharing what God has done for me with many people. I envision having a place where people can come and be renewed.

Bibliography

1. Kopans et al, The New England Journal of Medicine, vol.310 No 15, Breast Imaging; 1984

2. Haskell, C.M. and Casciato, D.A; *Breast Cancer;* 2000.

3. Gregory, Dr. David M. and Russell, Dr. Cynthia K; *Cancer Stories on Life and Suffering;* McGill Queens University Press; 1999

4. Henderson, C; *Hematology and Oncology;* Chapter 319, Breast Cancer.

5. Bosworth, FF; *Christ the Healer;* Fleming H Revell Publishing, 2000.

6. Austin and Hitchcock; *Breast Cancer; What You Should Know (But May Not Be Told),* 1994

7. Wadler, J; *My Breast;* Addison-Wesley Publishing Company; 1992

8. D'Adamo; *Eating Right for Your Type;* GP Putnam's Sons, New York, 1996

9. Plant, Jane A; *Your Life in Your Hands;* Thomas Dunne Books, New York, 2001.

10. Kradjian, R.M; *Save Yourself From Breast Cancer;* Berkely Publishing Group, 1994

11. Siegle, Bernie; *Peace, Love and Healing;* Harper Perennial, 1998.

12. Day, Lorraine, M.D; *You Can't Improve on God* (video), Rockford Press, 2000.

13. Colbert, Don, M.D; *The Bible Cure For Cancer;* Siloam Press, 1999.

14. Dufty, William; *Sugar Blues,* Warner Books Edition, 1975.

15. Day, Lorraine, M.D; *Sorting Through the Maze of Alternative Medicine* (video), Rockford Press, 2000

16. Malkmus, Rev.George; *God's Way to Ultimate Health,* Hallelujah Acres Publishing; 1995.

17. Walker, Norman W; *Fresh Vegetable and Fruit Juices;* Norwalk Press; 1978, Published annually since 1936.

18. Perkins, John; *A Presciption For Life;* ProMotion Publishing; 1997.

19. Batmanghelidj, F, MD.; *Your Body's Many Cries For Water;* Global Health Solutions; 1997.

20. Malkmus, George; *Why Christians Get Sick;* Treasure House Edition, 1995.

21. Diamond, Harvey; *You Can Prevent Breast Cancer;* ProMotion Publishing, 1995.

22. Newman, Laura; *Make Your Juicer Your Drug Store;* Benedict Lust Publications; 1992.

23. White, Ellen G.; *Ministry of Healing;* Better Living Publications; 2000.

24. Robbins, John; *Diet For a New World;* Avon Books Inc; 1993.

25. Young, Robert O. Ph.D. and Shelley; *The pH Miracle;* Warner Books Inc; 2002.

26. Klaper, Dr. Michael; *A Diet For All Reasons* (video); Michael Klaper M.D. Nutritional Services; 1992.

27. Jensen, Dr. Bernard; *A New Lifestyle for Health and Happiness;* Bernard Jensen Enterprizes; 1980

28. White, Ellen G; *Counsels on Diet and Foods;* The Ellen G White Estate; 1976.

29. *Hallelujah Testimonies 2* (video); Hallelujah Acres; 1999.

30. Jensen, Bernard, D.C. Ph.D.; *Rejuvenation and Regeneration;* Bernard Jensen Publisher; 1988.

31. Jensen, Bernard, PhD; *Nutrition Handbook, Book#1;* Bernard Jensen Publisher; 1993.

32. Jensen, Bernard, PhD; *Forever Young Living, Handbook #2;* Bernard Jensen Publisher; 1998.

33. Meyerowitz, Steve; *Wheatgrass, Nature's Finest Healer,* Sproutman Publications, 6th edition, 1999

34. McNeilus, Mary Ann, MD; *God's Healing Way;* Mercy Valley Farm; 1998.

35. *Alternative Medicine magazine; "Good Fish, Bad Fish";* p 41; Dorothy Foltz-Gray; May, 2003.

36. *Alternative Medicine magazine; "Good Fish, Bad Fish";* p 42; Dorothy Foltz-Gray; May, 2003.

37. *Environmental Health Perspectives doi;* 10; 1289/ehp.5754

38. DeKramer, Connie and Bill; *Cooking for Health Organically;* Issue No.6; p 4; June 2003.

39. *The World Book Encyclopedia;* Volume 3; World Book-Childcraft International, Inc; Copyright 1980.

40. Baker-Laporte, Paula; Elliott, Erica; Banta, John; *Prescriptions for A Healthy House;* New Society Publishers; Second Printing June 2002.

41. Northrup, Dr. Christiane; *The Wisdom of Menopause;* Bantam Books; March, 2003

42. Diamond, John, M.D; *Your Body Doesn't Lie;* Warner Books, Inc; Copyright, 1979.

43. Walker, Dr. Norman; *Colon Health;* Norwalk Press; Printed annually since 1979, 1995 edition.

44. Malkmus, Rhonda; *Recipes for Life from God's Garden;* Hallelujah Acres Publishing; Copyright, 1998

45. Howell, Dr. Edward; *Enzyme Nutrition, The Food Enzyme Concept;* Copyright, 1985, Edward Howell.

46. Wright, Dr. Jonathan V; *Nutrition and Healing,* Vol 10, issue 2; Feb 2003.

47. Swope, Mary Ruth; *Listening Prayer;* Springdale: Whitaker House; 1987

48. Carter, Albert E; *The Cancer Answer; National Institute of Reboundology;* Copyright 1988.

49. Walker, Dr. Norman; *Water can Undermine Your Health;* Copyright 1974 by Dr. N. W. Walker; Edited and revised 1995.

50. Kroeger, Hanna; *Cancer Traditional and New Concepts;* Compiled by Hanna Kroeger; Chapel of Miracles; No publication date listed; ISBN: 1-883713-06-4

51. Head, Kathleen A; *Estriol: Safety and Efficacy;* Alternative Medicine Review Volume 3, Number 2; 1998.